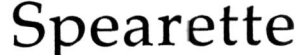

Spearette

To my daughters
Kate & Anne
and my grandchildren
Emilie, Tom, Jessica, Alice & Sophie

Spearette

A personal account of
the Hadfield–Spears Ambulance
Unit
1940–1945

by
Rachel Millet

Fern House

First published in 1998 by

Fern House

General Non-fiction Publishers

High Street   Haddenham   ELY   Cambs   CB6 3XA

ISBN 0 9524897 3 2

A catalogue record for this book
is available from the British Library

Jacket by Chris Winch Design
Printed and bound by The Basingstoke Press (75) Limited

SPEARETTE

A memoir of the Hadfield–Spears Ambulance Unit

When the Second World War broke out Rachel Millet (*née* Howell-Evans), a qualified children's nurse, was head matron at a boys' preparatory school. France fell, and she decided to join the Mechanised Transport Corps as a driver. Hearing that the Hadfield–Spears Hospital – somewhere in the Middle East with the Free French forces – needed drivers, she applied and was accepted.

Spearette (the French nickname for a Hadfield–Spears girl) tells the story of Rachel Millet's adventures as driver and nurse with the Hospital. Having travelled across the desert with the Eighth Army, and through Italy, she became an honorary Commando to land on the south coast of France preparatory to the main invasion.

Spearette is an intensely immediate and exciting story, with a distressing ending as the petulant General de Gaulle peremptorily ordered the Hospital to be disbanded because the crowds at the Paris Victory Parade dared to cheer: 'Vive Spears!'

CONTENTS

Glossary

1   Joining the Circus   1

2   El Alamein   17

3   Life in the Desert   29

4   The Longest Convoy Drive   37

5   Victory in North Africa   51

6   Return to Tunisia   61

7   On to Italy   68

8   Across the Garigliano River   81

9   To Rome and the Vatican   92

10   The Great Adventure   103

11   Arrival in France   113

12   Forward Unit to Lyons   128

13   Lyons   139

14   Home Leave   150

15   Alsace   164

16   The Last Battle   176

Supplement   191

GLOSSARY

ACL	Ambulance Chirurgicale Légère – provided ambulances and first aid
Alex	Alexandria
atelier lourd	heavy mechanical workshop attached to the Regiment
ATS	Auxiliary Territorial Service
au poil	by a hair's breadth
BIMP	Bataillon d'Infanterie de Marine et du Pacifique (Pacific Infantry Division)
Le Boudin	Black Pudding – song of the Foreign Legion
CB	Confined to Barracks
CCS	Casualty Clearing Station
les Chasseurs Alpins	Alpine Riflemen
le deuxième bureau	the intelligence department
en mission	on detached service
FAU	Friends' Ambulance Unit
felucca	narrow lateen-rigged vessel of the Mediterranean
fellah	Arab peasant (plural: *fellahin*)
FFI	*Maquis* (The French Resistance)
fusilier marin	Marine
le génie	equivalent to British sapper (Royal Engineer)

gestionnaire	administrator
GMC	a heavy transport vehicle
GOSH	Great Ormond Street Hospital for Sick Children
goum	Arab contingent
goumier	Arab scout
les grands blessés	the seriously wounded
HCM	Hôpital Chirurgical Militaire
HQ	headquarters
khamseen, khamsin	hot, southerly wind blowing March to May, especially in Egypt
LCM	landing craft (mechanised)
leaguer	an encampment
le train	transport
l'intendance	supplies administration
maison de retraite	old people's home
marionette	soldiers' name for French auxiliary nurses
matériel	equipment
milice	militia
MTC	Mechanised Transport Corps
NAAFI	Navy, Army and Air Force Institutes
Nannies	nickname for hospital sisters
pinard	wine
Popote des Officiers	Officers' Mess

PoW	prisoner of war
QA	Queen Alexandra's (Royal Army Nursing Corps – QARANC, or Royal Naval Nursing Corps – QARRNS)
RASC	Royal Army Service Corps
redcap	military policeman
REME	Royal Electrical and Mechanical Engineers
sapper	military engineer, member of the Royal Engineers
service sanitaire	hospital service
le service de santé	medical service
SHAEF	Supreme Headquarters Allied Expeditionary Force
sous officier	non-commissioned officer
Spearette	French nickname for a Hadfield–Spears girl
tarbush	fez-like cap, usually red with a silk tassel, worn by Muslim men alone or as part of a turban
tirailleur	black African serviceman (sharp-shooter, sniper)
transmissions	wireless, *etc*
VAD	Voluntary Aid Detachment
Very light	(to rhyme with query) coloured signalling flare fired from a special pistol, especially at sea, named after Edward W Very, US naval ordnance officer
wadi	a dried-out river bed. When it rains – which, thankfully, happens in the Western desert only at the end of the winter –wadis become raging torrents, carrying anything in their way down to the sea
YWCA	Young Women's Christian Association

1

JOINING THE CIRCUS

When the Second World War was declared, I was on holiday from my job as head matron at a boys' preparatory school in Northamptonshire. I had spent three years qualifying as a sick children's nurse at Great Ormond Street Hospital and this was my first post. I had already decided that two years at the school was long enough and was thinking of a change of scenery. The outbreak of war gave me my change; I gave in my notice and appeased the headmaster by finding a replacement – a friend who had qualified with me at GOS. I joined the VADs and was sent to the military hospital at Tidworth. I hoped to follow in the footsteps of one of my aunts who had served in France as a VAD in the First World War.

When France fell, I realised that this was not going to happen so my friend Biddy Pattinson and I decided to join the Mechanised Transport Corps, a voluntary women's corps which provided drivers anywhere they were required. The MTC gave us a stringent driving test, which happily we both passed. We then spent the next three weeks training at their headquarters near Sloane Square and living in state in a large house in Portland Place owned by one of Biddy's cousins.

We were drilled and marched through the streets of London by a ferocious sergeant from the Brigade of Guards. We were taught first aid, map reading and car maintenance. At the end of three weeks we were given exams and 'passed out' as lieutenants. We were given a few days' leave to buy our uniform, which we had to pay for ourselves, and were then posted to the Port of London. Here, for the next six months, we drove a variety of vehicles – ambulances, food canteens, lorries and cars – around the East India Docks.

We shared a comfortable air-raid shelter with sitting room, bedroom and bathroom with two other MTC drivers, each pair working 48 hours on and 48 hours off. We were fed by the Port of London Authority, mostly on conger eels, which were quite revolting. We enjoyed our work and would probably have spent the rest of the War there if we had not heard through the grapevine that the Hadfield–Spears Hospital, somewhere in the Middle East with the Free French forces, had asked the MTC for four replacement drivers. We knew nothing about the hospital or the Free French forces but the thought of action abroad was too good an opportunity to miss and we immediately put our names down. We went for an interview with

Dorea Stanhope, Lady Spears' representative in England, who had the task of choosing replacement drivers and sisters for the Hospital. We were lucky enough to be picked.

Dorea gave us a long list of tropical equipment to buy and pay for ourselves – camp bed, drill uniform, tin trunk, sleeping bag, topee, *etc*. We also had to collect identity papers and an identity disc, establishing our new status, French and military, and be vetted by security. The Ministry of Information gave us bundles of propaganda leaflets to be disposed of *en route*.

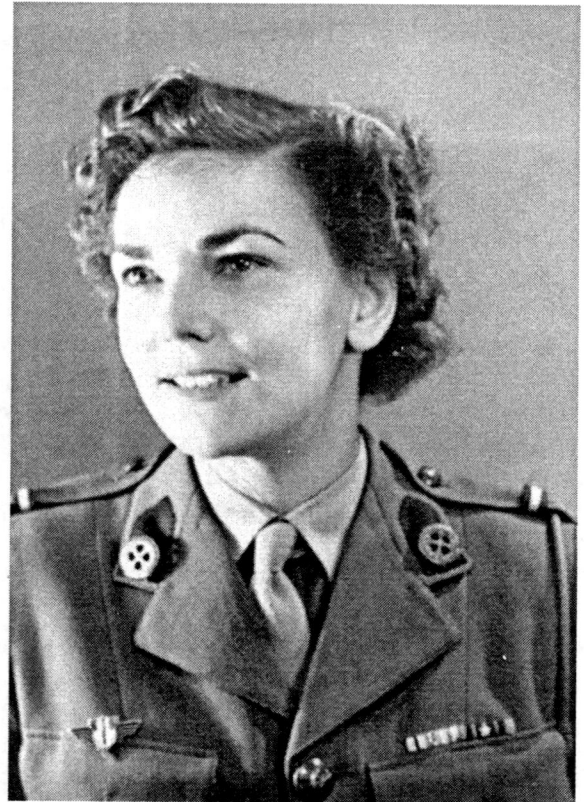

The author.

Biddy and I continued to work in the Port of London until the end of February 1942 when Dorea told us to prepare to leave. It was frustrating having nothing to do and there were many false alarms until at long last, in May, we received our marching orders. Dorea telephoned and said she would meet us on platform 2 at Olympia Station at 8pm the following day.

I don't know who was the more relieved, me or my parents who had never ceased to criticise me for leaving the VADs. I could not get away quickly enough. My father gave me the compass and binoculars he had had in the Middle East in the First World War.

My uniform and equipment was all packed and all we had to do was to catch the first train to London. I spent the night with my two maiden aunts in their flat near Sloane Square. (They were both killed later in the war by one of the first doodlebugs to fall on London.)

Biddy's mother came up with her and I met them both the next morning at Portland Place. We spent the morning packing our suitcases for the cabin and repacking our tin trunks with items 'not wanted on voyage'. We strapped together our flea-bags, camp beds, canvas buckets and felt-covered water bottles. Various friends and relations had given us a miscellaneous collection of 'useful' presents, including cotton lavatory-seat covers (against VD), woollen stomach protectors (against chills), and purses attached to belts to be worn under our clothes in case we were robbed! Needless to say we never used any of them.

Dorea was waiting at the station for us; the rest of our party turned up one by one and we were introduced to one another. When we had all assembled she took her 'flock' to the Officer OC Troops who assigned us a carriage.

It was still dark when we arrived next morning at the port, which we learnt was Greenock. We were given mugs of hot sweet tea and a bun on the platform and separated into two groups – men on one side, women on the other – then into respective units. We were much the smallest and least known but as we were ranked as officers no one was in charge of us, which was a blessing. After some delay we were taken to the quayside and embarked immediately on an impressive French liner, the *Pasteur*, France's newest flagship of the Messinger Maritime. She had been carrying a cargo of American war material destined for France, and re-routed to England on de Gaulle's orders. She had been hurriedly changed into a troop ship and most of her luxury fittings removed. It was rumoured that we had 5,500 troops on board who were being rushed to the Middle East to replace casualties. We were met at the top of the gangway by OC Troops who gave us the number of our cabin. The six of us were allotted a spacious cabin with three-tiered bunks on either side, a wash basin at one end, a dressing table at the other, a chest of drawers and a cupboard, enough for our clothes and belongings – one drawer each, so we had to be tidy.

The other women in uniform were squashed as many as ten to a cabin the same size as ours. We were told to tidy ourselves up and go down to the dining room for breakfast. What a meal – a choice of five or more cooked dishes, toast, marmalade, as much butter as we wanted, fruit, coffee or tea and even porridge. After British rations we could hardly believe our eyes. Much refreshed, we returned to our cabin, unpacked, sorted out where each of us should sleep and divided up the hanging space and drawers. We were fairly cramped but no one complained.

We also started to get to know one another: five replacement drivers and one sister, Jean Williams, who had been with the hospital in France and been left behind when they sailed for the Middle East because of illness. Westminster Hospital trained, Jean was blue-eyed, brown haired and very pretty, popular with staff and patients alike, and a most efficient nurse who before long became Head Sister. She was also great fun and ready for anything and we became great friends.

Iris Goodwin was small, neat and tidy. She came from a very devoted family; her mother was the lynch-pin as her father, a parson, had died quite young. Iris was always ready to undertake any job, however unpleasant, and never got drawn into the rows or disagreements which sometimes occurred. She also became a very good friend; we did a lot of driving and had many adventures together. I saw a lot of her after the war until her tragic death from cancer when she was only forty. Biddy, Jean, Iris and I made up a foursome and spent most of our time together. The two other drivers were Ruth Nicholls and Aimee Potter. Ruth left us soon after our arrival at the hospital. We learnt later that she had joined the unit as a means of reaching the Middle East where her brother was a general at Headquarters; he found her an easier job as a secretary.

We set sail at 12.30pm on 9 May 1942. The huge ship slowly left the quayside, turned round with the help of tugs looking like small terriers, and made her way majestically down the Clyde. When she reached the estuary and the open sea we saw that it was thick with ships of every description: fishing boats, tugs, motor boats, submarines, corvettes, destroyers, cruisers, battleships and troopships. We watched, fascinated, while our convoy mustered. We set off down the North Sea, merchant ships and troop ships guarded by several destroyers and a battle cruiser *The Golden Sovereign*. It reminded me of a flock of sheep flanked by sheepdogs.

It was very exciting watching signals being flashed from ship to ship but alarming too, wondering where exactly we were going, how long our voyage would take, and whether we would be torpedoed or shipwrecked. I was worried that I would be sea sick but I wasn't. For me it was a great adventure; the first time I had been out of England, and escaped from the iron discipline of my parents. I may have felt apprehensive but I don't think that I was frightened.

Unlike the ATS, WAAFs and Queen Alexandra sisters, who were drilled and under orders at all times, we had no duties and were under no one's orders, except for boat drill – which could happen at any time of day or night; we never knew whether or not it was for real. We were all given Mae West life jackets which we had to keep with us wherever we were. If the alarm was sounded, we had to be on the correct deck and lined up by our allotted lifeboat within so many minutes; we got a rocket if we were late. The crew of each lifeboat practised getting it afloat but I am glad to say we never had to get in.

There was plenty to do on board ship – gymnastics and keep-fit sessions, deck tennis and quoits, a well-stocked library and dancing in the evenings. We made friends with army and naval officers and Biddy and I played bridge most evenings after dark. I spent a lot of time on deck watching the convoy manoeuvre as it sailed along.

Travelling with us were several Frenchmen on their way to join Free French forces and a General and Madame d'Assonville, who were the bane of our lives. Although she had no right to do so, as we all had officer rank, Madame insisted on censoring our letters. To get our own back we collected all the dirty stories we could find and sent them to fictitious addresses in England. She also tried to get us under her husband's orders, but in this she failed. An officer from the Foreign Legion, Captaine La Baume, gave Iris and me lessons in French grammar and conversation. He was so nice and we were so hopeless; I think he was in despair by the time we reached Durban.

We reached Durban after three weeks at sea. Mersa Matruh had fallen and there seemed to be some doubt about where we should be sent; as a result we spent two happy weeks in Durban. The six of us were billeted in a small hotel near the sea. We thought the food was marvellous: huge breakfasts and a variety of fruit that we had never eaten before – avocados, passion fruit, guavas and many others.

Durban was a town of many different races, all living in separate, well-defined areas. There was no apartheid then and we were quite ignorant of any tension. Natal was originally a British settlement so most of the 'whites' were of English descent; I don't remember meeting any Boers. There were a great many Indians who worked mainly in hotels, shops and on taxis. The chief native tribe was Zulu; Zulus also drove taxis and pulled rickshaws with a fine disregard for other traffic. They were dressed in clothes of brilliant colours, skins and feathers with strings of beads around their necks and ankles and head-dresses of bright feathers. They also carried spears, shields and knives. They were tall and long-legged and their feet hardly touched the ground as they sped along with their rickshaws.

All the South Africans we met were very friendly and welcoming and did their best to entertain us. We were given free tickets to cinemas and the theatre, invited to their homes, offered horses to ride and taken on sight-seeing trips to the Valley of a Thousand Hills and along the coast. There seemed to be no shortage of anything, no rationing or coupons; everything, including petrol, was plentiful and cheap.

Most of the friends we had made on the *Pasteur* had left Durban by the time we embarked on to an old and battered Union Castle ship. We met up with a new lot of army personnel, several officers from the Sudanese army, VADs, QAs and ATS odds and ends on their way to join their regiments. We were squashed together in a much smaller cabin than on the *Pasteur*, with very little room to move or put our belongings. When we reached the Red Sea the ship stopped; it was like a furnace. The women were given a corner on the top deck and allowed to sleep up there. It was much cooler there than below deck and there was an occasional welcome breeze. We shared showers with the other women; there was only salt water and we were given special salt-water soap to wash ourselves and our clothes in. It did not lather like ordinary soap and we never felt really clean. We all suffered from prickly heat – rather like eczema and very irritating. We never stopped sweating and the prickly heat was worse wherever there was pressure – around our waists, inside knees and elbows – and even in our hair. The itching drove us mad. Powder was said to help, but as we were permanently drenched with sweat it soon washed off. We hung towels round our necks to wipe off the surplus moisture. We were always thirsty. All alcohol and fresh water ran out after our first week sitting in the Red Sea and we had only desalted water from the ship's condensers, which did not taste very nice. Someone said that after three cups of tea one ceased to sweat for a while, but not for long. We sweated so much that we did not need to urinate. This seemed to worry the men much more than the women; I went for two days without passing a drop. To prevent heat-stroke we were ordered to eat two tablespoonfuls of salt each day to replace the salt we lost.

After two weeks sitting still in the heat of the Red Sea our Captain was given permission to berth at Massawa in Eritrea. We were in a pretty poor state by now; several of the crew and passengers, including two QAs, were suffering from heat-stroke and were flown to the cooler heights of Addis Abbaba where they were admitted to hospital. The ship's stokers, buried in the depths of the ship, suffered the most and two of them died.

We were allowed off the ship for the two days we were at Massawa, but had to return at nightfall. The British Consul was very kind to us and kept open house. He allowed us to use his bathroom and plied us with drink telling us that, to survive the heat of Eritrea, alcohol was essential and that teetotallers lasted no time at all out there. There was nothing much to see at Massawa. Along the coast there were large salt pans and not much else. It was too hot to go walkabout. After Massawa we continued our journey. No more sitting motionless in the Red Sea and with the ship re-stocked with fresh water and alcohol. Three days later we docked at Suez. The smells and yells of Egypt, which were to become so familiar to us, hit us for the first time. The smell of Egypt is unique: a mixture of camel dung, drains, spices, attar of roses and hashish found nowhere else in the world. The cries of 'Baksheesh', and other yells to which we were to become accustomed resounded around the quayside.

We packed our belongings from our cabin, all clearly labelled 'Hadfield–Spears', then threw the topees overboard (they had caused us so much embarrassment on the ship as they were fifty years out of date). We also disposed of the ridiculous pamphlets given to us by the Ministry of Information in London – who did they think we would give them to and where? Having got rid of our surplus possessions we waited on deck with our luggage for our instructions and watched the ship being unloaded. We were dismayed by our non-existent disembarkation orders. No one knew anything about us, or had any orders for us. The OC Troops at the quayside said that he thought the Hospital was in Syria but he was not sure and that we had better get on the train to Cairo, find ourselves lodgings for the night and contact the Free French the following morning. We were loaded on to the train along with our luggage and off we went. We were all very disheartened; none of us had any Egyptian money, nor could we speak a word of Egyptian. We had no knowledge of Cairo, its streets or hotels. Once again, it was pitch dark when we arrived. We were lucky to find several military police on the platform who helped us find our luggage and changed some of our English money into piastres. They found us two taxis and gave us a list of hotels and their addresses. We must have gone to at least a dozen hotels before we found one which would take us in; it was very seedy and had only one room for the six of us, but we were so depressed and frightened that we accepted it thankfully.

A few days after we arrived, Lady Spears flew in from Beirut where her husband, General Sir Louis Spears, was a British representative in the Lebanon and Syria. She had come to inspect the new arrivals, and took the trouble to get to know us by allowing each of us to drive her. Lady Spears was the Directress or La Générale (her husband being a general) but we referred to her as 'The Gee'. She had to spend most of her time in Beirut but kept a keen control over the Hospital and visited us as often as she could and whenever she was needed.

It's difficult for me to write about Lady Spears as we became great friends after the war. I admired her more than anyone else I knew and she was fond of me. She was rather strange in appearance; I imagine she must have been between 50 and 60 years old when I joined the unit and was therefore much older than anyone else. She was heavily made up with mascara smudged down her eyes and lipstick smudged over her mouth. She had a wavering husky voice and a slight head tremor. I have been told that she was almost beautiful when she was young, and she still had beautiful grey eyes.

Her father, owner of Borden's Milk, had been a very rich man. She was devoted to him; he died when she was about eighteen, and her mother took her on a round-the-world trip to help her recover from her grief. In India she met an English missionary to whom her mother married her off. They lived a very simple life with few luxuries or entertainments. She happened to be back in England when the 1914 war started and was enjoying herself for the first time in her life when she realised that she was a rich woman. She decided she would not return to India and instead offered her services and money to Madame de la Panouse, Head of the French Red Cross in England and wife of the French Military Attaché, General de la Panouse, an Anglophile who had spent years in England. Madame de la Panouse thought that she was just another spoilt American with more money than sense and sent her to one of the worst field hospitals in France – mostly medical cases of typhoid, typhus and pneumonia, no trained nurses, no proper medical equipment, only squalor. She ended the war with a 100-bedded hospital, fully staffed and equipped, paid for entirely by herself. General Spears, British Liaison Officer with the French, turned up at her hospital one day *en mission*. She told me she suffered a *coup de foudre* – they fell in love immediately and she sent her husband a cable telling him she was getting a divorce. He cabled back 'do nothing until I arrive' but by the time he was able to get a passage back she had divorced him and married Spears. When I asked her one day what her first husband was like she replied: 'My dear, he was so insignificant that I can't remember'. During the USA depression her brother lost all her money. Undeterred, she started to write novels under her maiden name – Mary Borden. They were very successful; two at least were made into films and chosen as 'book of the month' by the Book Society. With the money they made she bought a cottage near Ascot and paid for the education of their only child, Michael. Spears in the meantime became an MP, among other things, and wrote a very successful book called *Liaison Officer*.

When the Second World War broke out Lady Spears (financed by Lady Hadfield) offered a fully-equipped field hospital to the French. They were based at St Jean le Bassel in Lorraine and escaped to Bordeaux, one hop in front of the Germans advancing across France. They had to leave all their cars and equipment behind when they reached Bordeaux, catching one of the last boats to leave for England. Back again in England, Lady Spears set about equipping her third hospital. She could no longer count on any help from Lady Hadfield who was unable to escape from her villa in the South of France. She sent an SOS to a friend in the USA – Mrs Benson – who was Head of the British and French War Relief and who sent her £20,000, enough to pay for all she needed. She recruited sufficient nurses and drivers to make up the strength as before. She offered her services to General de Gaulle who had been helped out of France by General Spears – Spears had lent him his aeroplane – and off they went to join the First Free French Brigade somewhere in the Middle East.

On its arrival in the Middle East, the hospital was sent to Syria. They nursed many casualties during the bitter fighting between the Vichy French and the Free French. When that war was ended, they and the Free French Brigade joined the Eighth Army and were stationed at various places including Tobruk and Timini.

When the French Brigade was at Bir Hakim, the hospital sent a forward unit from Tobruk. Kit Tatham Warner and Rosaleen Forbes took it in turns to keep contact with them and Kit was there the day before Bir Hakim fell. When we returned to Tobruk and the war had advanced to Tunisia, Kit spent a lot of time trying to find her old dug-out, without success. All she found was someone's discarded thigh bone – she presumed an amputation. When Bir Hakim fell they raced back to the Delta, one of the few units with all the equipment intact. They were sent first to Ikingo camp and then to the unbearably hot and dusty Kilo 4 on the Cairo-en-Suez road. In July they moved into an empty school in Heliopolis, which is where we joined them.

Lady Spears wrote a full account of their time in Syria and their journey and adventures up and down the desert in her book *Journey Down A Blind Alley* published after the end of the war. She had endless battles – which she always won – with the British Generals who insisted that no women were allowed in the desert.

The tented hospital consisted of five surgical wards, each with 25 beds, and two medical wards each with 20 beds. There was sufficient bed linen for 200 beds in all – mattresses, pillows, sheets, pale blue blankets, mosquito nets and pyjamas – so that each wounded patient could be stripped of his bloodstained and torn uniform before being washed and dressed in clean pyjamas and put to bed between the clean white sheets. As a field hospital, it was unique.

The hospital was completely mobile. We had 60 vehicles: ten five-ton lorries, four water buggies, ambulances, a mobile operating theatre and our five staff cars: four Fords and one Chevrolet. The theatre tents were equipped with four hydraulic operating tables and lit by powerful operating lamps run from their own generators. Two dozen sterilising drums packed with surgical instruments provided everything necessary for all operations, including dentistry and ophthalmic surgery. The hospital was as self-sufficient as it was possible for a mobile casualty hospital to be. It had its own X-ray truck equipped with tables and dark-room and its own dentistry, pharmacy and bacteriology departments.

The sisters, when on duty, wore pretty blue dresses and blue cloaks; out of uniform they wore battle dress as we did, or drill skirts and khaki blouses. We only wore our MTC uniform for inspections by generals or on special occasions. We all wore desert boots, which were more practical against the heat of the sand when the temperature was 30°F or more – and they kept the sand out of our feet.

Colonel Vernier was head of the hospital under Lady Spears. He was the son of a French Protestant missionary; his father had spent a lot of time in Tahiti and had looked after the dying Gauguin. Colonel Vernier was a regular army doctor. His wife and children were in France; his wife was an invalid and died during the war; the children were then looked after by his parents and school-teacher brother. Colonel Vernier was a very jolly man, full of enterprise, universally liked and respected – and a brilliant surgeon.

The second surgeon, Captain Thibaux, was also an army doctor and an excellent surgeon who became a good friend. The third surgeon was Coupigny; very good looking. He became a great friend of Iris; we always thought they would marry after the war, but it was not to be.

The Chief Medical Officer, Captain Jibery, was second in command to Vernier. He had changed his name to protect his wife and children living in Normandy. He was rather aloof and no one knew him well. When I worked in the Hospital I had several differences of opinion with him and blamed him for the death of a legionnaire who was very ill with dysentery. I wanted to give the patient a blood transfusion but Jibery said it was unnecessary. The soldier suddenly collapsed and by the time Jibery agreed to give him a transfusion it was too late.

Lieutenant Aboucher was Syrian and was the only dentist when I joined the unit. His drill was worked by a pedal, like an old-fashioned sewing machine. He liked to chat while he was working and I remember sitting in the dental chair outside his tent in the desert having a molar stopped. His drill would get slower and slower and eventually stop as he was carried away by the latest gossip.

Our second dentist, Captain Prochesson, joined the Hospital much later. He was a brilliant dental surgeon as well, and achieved amazing results by wiring up broken jaws and facial bones. He disappeared whenever the Division went into action and took part in the attack with, I think, the artillery. His only child, a boy of six years old, was killed and his wife seriously wounded by German Stukas machine gunning refugees on the road from Paris. In this way he was avenging them.

Lieutenant Salamon, known as 'Solly', Jew and Rabbi from Palestine, was our number two physician. He was fat, jolly and cuddly and everyone's favourite. As well as looking after our medical patients he was in charge of the VD ward. He gave us lessons about the Jewish religion, the significance of the Passover *etc*, and he officiated at the burials of Jewish soldiers.

Pierre Mergier, one of the youngest officers, was the Head Pharmacist. He was very nice and kind; his family lived at Neuilly in Paris and were incredibly kind, keeping open house to all of us whenever we were there. His younger brother joined us when we were in Alsace.

Aspirant Schick, also Jewish, was in the middle of his training as a doctor; he helped in the theatre and anywhere else he was needed.

Lieutenant Aurès was the gestionnaire when we arrived. He was replaced by Lieutenant Duprez when we were in Tunis. Sergeant Yantze, an Argentinean, was in charge of the X-ray equipment. He was a trained photographer and was always taking photographs.

We had two padres. Père Boileau was the RC Chaplain; until the war broke out he had been in a monastery in Bulgaria. He was also in charge of the rations for the officers' mess, so we were frequently ordered to drive him around the countryside in Italy and France – and even in the desert, where he succeeded in buying tunny and figs to supplement our army rations. He was very short tempered when things went wrong; otherwise he was friendly to us. He was also a very good and enthusiastic amateur photographer. Père Bonjour was the Protestant chaplain, we saw very little of him and I hardly knew him at all.

There were thirty French and North African non-commissioned officers and some seventy soldiers from French Equatorial Africa. There were two Syrian cooks: Amar, the head cook, was a cheery individual, and he and his assistant succeeded in producing a surprising variety of dishes based on bully beef and the monotonous British rations. Only the disgusting pilchards in tomato sauce defeated them. They had their own mobile kitchen and whenever we arrived tired and hungry after a long convoy drive they always had hot soup and thick sweet tea ready waiting for us. Amar was also one of Solly's most regular patients in the VD ward.

The Tirailleurs, most from Chad and Senegal, did all the heavy work in the hospital, carrying water, helping in the kitchens, washing the dirty ward linen, waiting in the mess and working as orderlies in the hospital wards. We had two orderlies for our own tents: Jean and Michel; they were marvellous, looked after us with devotion, were always in good humour and treated us as if we were their own children. They were very smart in their best uniform, with bright red cummerbunds made of yards and yards of flannel wound round their waists, and red kepis. When I fetched supplies from the NAAFI, I could not understand why they ordered so many tins of black boot polish until I happened to see Jean getting ready for a parade one day, polishing his legs and arms with polish until they shone like ebony.

The English personnel consisted of 38 Friends' Ambulance Unit personnel, and a fluctuating number of sisters and drivers, roughly six of each. The FAU was organised by the Quakers; Michael Rowntree (from the chocolate family) was in charge of them with Patrick Barr, his second in command. Michael had great tact, and understood the complexity of the Circus. He got on well with everyone and the Colonel thought the world of him. He did not have an easy job – there were only six Quakers in his team who held the same pacifist views as he did; the rest were conscientious objectors, with many different reasons for not fighting. They were from all walks of civilian life – several were artists, one was an Oxford don, Pat Barr was an actor. Two ended up as bishops after the war. They worked extremely hard, dug latrines, put up and took down all the tents, provided orderlies for the hospital wards, maintained and drove all the hospital vehicles (except for our staff cars), ran the electrical generators and worked in their own maintenance garage. They were willing to help and turn their hands to anything and were very kind in helping us with our cars when we asked them. I don't think we were always very nice to them, as several of us had friends or relations fighting in the forces and thought that they should be doing the same.

The five trained sisters when we arrived at Heliopolis were Jean Blair, Evelyn Fulroth, Edith Irving, Franka Kohen and Joan Hemingway.
Jean was older than most of us, very Scottish, small and wiry and rather prim. She left us when we were in Tunisia.
Evelyn, who had done her training at the Westminster Hospital with Jean, had also been with Lady Spears' first hospital in France. She was very pretty with deep blue eyes, fair hair and an English pink and white complexion. She was much admired for her looks as well as her efficiency as a nurse. She generally looked after any wounded officers we had. She married Jim Cottrell, one of the FAU, before the end of the war.
Edith was also older. She was rather prickly at times but a marvellous nurse and saved many lives, often staying up all night to give a severely wounded soldier special care. She had a subtle sense of humour which was always unexpected. When we were in the desert she suddenly asked for leave to get married and told us all about this glamorous officer who was in love with her. We collected some nice wedding presents for her and wished her luck. Two weeks later she was back; the officer had reneged on her. She never spoke about it and neither did we.
Franka was a Polish Jewess who had been training as a nurse in England at the outbreak of war. She was rather plump, fair haired, blue eyed and always worked in the operating theatre. She was

completely unflappable and fun to be with. All her family were killed by the Germans.

The drivers when we arrived were Jocelyn Russell, Kit Tatham Warner, Rosaleen Forbes, Barbara Graham, and Cynthia Toulmin.

Jocelyn was older than the rest of the drivers and married to an RAF officer who had been stationed in Cairo when she joined the Unit in January 1942. She admitted that her reason for joining was to be near him. Quite soon after she arrived he was posted to the Far East and she never saw him again; he was posted 'missing, presumed killed' when we were at Tobruk. All her letters to him were returned to her – which must have been dreadful, but she never broke down. She was good looking with sunburnished hair, a high colour and a good figure. She was always neat and tidy even in battle dress. She was very popular with the Division and we used to say 'more French than the French' as she spoke volubly, and made incredible *faux pas* which the French repeated with glee.

Kit was in charge of car maintenance and of the drivers' roster. I had known her and the rest of her family before the war. She was one of a large family of two brothers and five sisters and lived near my parents in Somerset. Her great love, like mine, was horses. She would ride anything lapped in a skin and was a fearless point-to-point rider before and after the war. She even rode a scatty mare which no one else could hold; it gave me three falls in one day's hunting, and gave Kit a crashing fall in a race.

Kit was also a first-class mechanic and taught us all how to clean out carburettors and petrol pumps and how to change half tracks and heavy desert tyres – she once made me change eight in one morning. She was small, fair and sturdily built, quite indomitable and completely fearless. She was also a bully and enjoyed bossing us around, often making us do unnecessary jobs.

Rosaleen Forbes – Rosie – spent part of her childhood in France and spoke perfect French; she knew and used all the swear words as well. She was dark haired and dark eyed and very pretty and was the youngest of us all. She celebrated her twenty-first birthday in the desert. A great favourite with everyone, she never got herself involved in any rows or disputes was always ready to volunteer for any unpleasant job. Lady Spears doted on her and when we first arrived she had been with her in Beyrouth as her driver.

Barbara arrived soon after we did. She had been with the hospital in France and in Syria and then left to do intelligence work in Tehran with Freya Stark – who, she told me, was extremely difficult to get on with. Barbara was delighted when May sent her an excuse to leave and take over from Jocelyn, who couldn't cope, as her representative with the Hospital. Barbara had auburn hair and a most delightful smile. She had been brought up in Cairo where her father had organised the entire water supply; her uncle, Russell Pasha, was a big noise in Egypt. She spoke French and Arabic and, like Kit, she was an excellent mechanic and had driven in motor rallies before the war. She was the opposite to meticulous Kit, never bothered much about her car and, when it conked out, got it going again with bits of string and wire and a kick in the right place.

It was through Barbara that we became friends with a Greek couple who lived in Alexandria: Kostia and Domina Rodocanachi. Domina lent us a car whenever we had a day off and Kostia presented an operating ambulance to the hospital fully equipped with the latest gadgets. They kept open house in their flat in Alexandria to all the women of the Unit, making us welcome with food and a bed.

Rosie and Cynthia had been friends before the war and had both been in France from the beginning. Cynthia left soon after we arrived to marry Peter Smith Dorien who, alas, was blown up in the King David Hotel at the end of the war, leaving Cynthia with a small daughter.

After the war I remained great friends with Barbara, Iris and Rosie, and of course with Biddy and Kit whom I had known before the war.

When we arrived, the hospital was installed in the Franco–Egyptian School at Heliopolis. We spent our first few days as drivers learning our way around the busy streets of Cairo and between the various units of the French Brigade encamped around the town.

The drivers were billeted in small empty rooms on the ground floor of the School. Biddy and I shared a room and I clearly remember our dismay at the lack of furniture and of all modern conveniences. Kit laughed and told us how lucky we were to be so gently initiated into the nomad life of the Unit. We had a roof over our heads, a stone floor under our feet and running water from a tap in the courtyard (even if it was cold), to say nothing of the civilisation of Cairo only a few miles away.

Biddy and I quickly learned all the tricks of making ourselves as comfortable as possible in whatever conditions: string stretched across the room or tent to hang clothes or washing from; orange boxes or, better still, ammunition boxes for tables and chairs; jerry cans, vastly superior to English petrol cans, for heating and storing water. Our tin trunks served as bedside tables. For the first time in my life I learned the meaning of the French phrase *démerdez vous*; untranslatable into polite English, it was to become our drivers' motto.

A few days after our arrival Lady Spears flew in from Syria to inspect her new recruits and to take charge. We took it in turns to drive her around in one of our staff cars. These cars were entirely our responsibility to service, maintain and keep clean and no one but us was allowed to drive them. They had already done a good mileage before we arrived and all but one survived to the end of the war, each clocking up more than 200,000 miles; there was very little left of their original components except their chassis. The cars were known by their numbers; the Fords were 64, 76, 82 and 91 and the Chevrolet (Marguerite) was 96. The Fords were all the same age and model. I started off with 64 and then changed to 82, which I kept until the end of the war. Iris had 76 for most of the war, Biddy 91 and Jocelyn 64. Rosie did not have a special car. Kit always drove and cared for the Chevrolet, known to the French as *La Belle Marguerite* from the time she sat outside Bir Hakim, nose down in a slit trench. Kit guarded her jealously but in fact no one else had the slightest desire to drive her and we moaned when we had to. That car was an absolute bitch, with a mind of her own. She always got there in the end, due to Kit's brilliance as a mechanic, but was guaranteed to do the unexpected and we all had scary drives in her. She was also extremely uncomfortable as Kit had fitted her with truck springs and she had to be weighed down with sand bags to keep her on the roads.

The first time I was detailed to drive Lady Spears I was very apprehensive as I had been told that she liked to be driven very fast and I was still learning my way around Cairo and its outskirts. When I asked her if this was true she laughed and told me to drive her at whatever speed I liked. When I got to know her better she proved to be the perfect passenger – as long as she was firmly ensconced in the back seat, where she would happily bounce up and down over the pot-holed roads engrossed in the latest detective story.

Lady Spears liked to get to her destination with the least possible delay, as did the Colonel, but as long as she was in the back she paid no attention to the route or near misses. If she was allowed into the seat next to the driver she was always convinced that she knew the best route and this led to wrong turnings and late arrivals. We were instructed that, in no circumstances whatsoever, was she to be allowed into the driving seat, as she was lethal.

The second time I drove 'The Gee' to Cairo we were travelling along one of the busy streets when, to my amazement, I suddenly saw a wheel which was obviously mine bowling along beside us. I managed to pull up beside the kerb without mishap and retrieve the wheel before it disappeared under the robe of an Egyptian. I had no idea what to do next, as the half-shaft had broken. The Gee was quite unperturbed; she suggested that I found her a taxi and then telephoned the hospital for assistance. This I did; Kit duly arrived with a breakdown lorry and I was ignominiously towed back to Heliopolis, hind wheels – or rather wheel – in the air. The next day Kit showed me how to replace a half shaft, one of the weak points of the Ford V8; that was why we usually carried a spare in the boot.

These first days at Heliopolis were very carefree. The Free French Brigade was resting and the hospital had only a few medical and accident cases. The drivers – nicknamed 'Spearettes' by the French – were not required to help in the wards and, at this stage, there was not a lot of driving for any of us. We were given a generous amount of time off and were able to go swimming, play tennis and ride at the Ghezera Sporting Club in Cairo, and to enjoy parties at the Cairo night clubs and hotels. We became good clients of Shepheard's and the Continental Hotels. We also learnt our way around the Brigade and got to know its various regiments. The First Armoured Division was part of the Eighth Army, and consisted amongst others of the 9th and 12th Lancers, the 10th Hussars and the Queen's Bays and Rifle Brigade. Kit, Biddy, Rosie and I all had friends in each, and Kit's eldest brother John was in the Queen's Bays.

Egypt itself fascinated me with her souks and mosques. The hot smell of horse and camel dung, mixed with the other potent smells of the Middle East, was exclusively Egyptian. It was a strange, exotic world of great riches and poverty: immaculate servants in immaculate uniforms, unforgettable food at Groppies and the Mohammed Ali Club. The Ghezera Sporting Club was, without doubt, the best in the world where every sport and game was played; there were also Shepheard's Hotel where 'one sat on the steps and watched the world go by', and a large choice of night clubs, each with its cabaret and belly dancers. Side by side with all this opulence was the extreme poverty of the poor, starving fellahin, tattered children with fly-encrusted eyes and open sores, emaciated horses and donkeys covered in weals and sores and everywhere beggars and the everlasting cry of 'Baksheesh'. The thieving, the bargaining, the fly whisks and tarbushes, the ever-present flies and bugs attacking indiscriminately the rich and the poor, the washed and the unwashed. Veiled women all in black, men smoking hubble-bubble pipes outside the cafés. Gully-gully men touting for customers to watch their tricks with snakes and chickens. Everywhere the British army, Redcaps looking for deserters and drunks, staff cars with flags flying rushing down the streets, soldiers on leave, soldiers on duty. The whole polyglot of race, creed and uniform. At this time Cairo must have been one of the most exciting cities in the world, however near or far Rommel and his army was, and he wasn't very far away.

2

EL ALAMEIN

Lady Spears left us at the beginning of August. On the fifteenth, we moved to Mena camp under the shadow of the Pyramids where we, the new girls, had our first experience of living in tents and sand – not realising at the time what a gentle introduction this was. We were still within driving distance of Cairo and close to the Pyramids Hotel, Mena House. We, the drivers, rented a permanent room at the Hotel for our days off where we could have a bath, wash our clothes, and sleep in comfort.

We were not the only inhabitants of Mena camp. Apart from our Brigade there were British and Indian regiments, including a regiment of Parsees. The latter put their dead on a high tower especially built for them, where the kites and vultures disposed of their bodies – a gruesome sight, and we were always afraid that one of the birds might drop a piece of flesh on our heads.

At Mena camp we learned to walk through sand and – more important – to drive through it without getting stuck. All our vehicles carried sand-tracks and we got no sympathy if we had to use them.

31 August 1942 – Rommel attacked the Eighth Army at Alam Halfa. Our Brigade was not engaged but as the battle flowed to and fro we sat in our cars and trucks with everything loaded up, leave cancelled, ready to do a quick flit if the worst happened and Rommel broke through the defences. Cairo was filled with smoke from the many bonfires of secret papers which the embassies burnt as a precaution but, luckily for everyone concerned, Rommel was held and after spending two or three days in our vehicles we unpacked again.

On 18 September we moved again, this time to Buseilli near the holy city of Rosetta on the banks of the Nile, where we waited for the Battle of El Alamein. A forward unit was sent up to the Free French Brigade which was in position in front of the escarpment of Himeimat, on the extreme left of the Eighth Army and near the Qattara depression.

On most days one of us would be detailed to drive up to the forward unit with rations, mail and medical supplies. I found it very exciting to be right up at the front line when no one knew when the attack would begin.

Back at the main hospital we prepared the full complement of 200 beds for the expected heavy casualties. Our hospital was housed in a series of Nissen huts next door to an Australian hospital, also housed in Nissen huts. We had proper wards, running water, showers, lavatories, sluice rooms and ward kitchens, and the compound included squash courts and even a cinema. In addition we each had a room to ourselves.

The Battle of El Alamein started at midnight on 23 October and ambulances started to arrive from the front the following evening. Lady Spears had arrived the day before and took charge of the hospital; the Colonel left for the forward unit immediately she arrived. He started operating almost at once on the wounded, who all passed through his hands before arriving at the main hospital.

Everyone worked flat out. I was put in charge of one of the surgical wards, Biddy and Iris worked in others and even Kit, who had never done a first aid or nursing course, helped with meals and blanket baths. Every bed in the hospital was soon filled and extra stretchers and camp beds were put up wherever there was a space.

My first experience of nursing wounded soldiers was very different from my Great Ormond Street training. My ward had forty beds in all, twenty on each side, and an instrument trolley in the centre. Each bed was made up with clean sheets and pillowcases, covered with bright blue blankets and with a locker for the soldier's personal belongings. I had an FAU orderly to help and two Senegalese to keep the ward clean and tidy.

To begin with I had to learn the French names for all the surgical instruments, medical equipment and so on and the French Army slang for various utensils – eg pistolet for urinal – not words one learnt in the school room. I also learnt a great deal about courage and the will to live and the wish to die.

Above all I had to learn to cope with horrendous wounds without showing faintness or distress. Luckily I was so busy I had not time to think of myself. Bullets made a small entry wound and a large exit, often taking with them pieces of clothing or anything else that stood in their way. Shrapnel made terrible jagged wounds. Landmines shattered arms and legs, and often blinded as well. Some of the saddest cases were men who had lost their eyes and hands through stepping on a mine. We prayed they would die, but they seldom did. The worst wounds to dress were amputations, often double. They took ages and caused agonising pain however careful one was. We gave morphia before we did them but it did not seem to help much.

Occasionally I helped out in the operating theatre when the Colonel was operating and Franka had a break. Wartime surgery was very different from what I had learnt at Great Ormond Street; amputations were never stitched up, a flap was left and the final operation was performed at a base hospital.

Badly infected wounds were sometimes put into plaster and maggots introduced which consumed all the putrefied flesh and left the wound clean and ready to be stitched up. We never told the men about the maggots as they would have been horrified. They used to complain of itchiness around the wound and we would say it was because it was healing.

Whenever the Colonel operated on a German he made a cross of Lorraine somewhere on his body. After each abdominal operation (whatever the nationality of the patient) he poured a whole can of ether into the abdominal cavity before he closed it which I found extraordinary, but it certainly worked.

The final casualties in the Brigade were heavy. The Foreign Legion in particular suffered great losses which included their Colonel, Dimitri Amilakvari, a Georgian prince and a legendary figure, beloved by his officers and men alike. He died in the ambulance bringing him to the hospital.

John Tatham Waters was killed in his tank; Kit and I quartered the desert after the battle was over, looking for his grave, but we never found it.

By 11 November the main attack was over and the greater part of the Brigade was pulled out of the line, leaving only the BIMP – an infantry regiment of Colonial troops and a regiment of Moroccan Spahis – to continue the chase with the Eighth Army. The Colonel packed up his forward unit and returned to us.

The wounded slowly recovered and were evacuated to convalescent homes or to specialist hospitals in Cairo. Here they were fitted with false limbs or underwent plastic surgery. A great many of our wounded were returned to their units fit and well.

As the work in the hospital wards decreased we returned to driving our cars again. One day I drove Lady Spears to the forward unit to visit the Colonel after the Eighth Army had finally broken through the German lines. We passed several prisoner of war camps, hastily constructed, full of prisoners and more trudging wearily along the roads, German and Italian. They looked like prisoners the world over – unshaven, bedraggled and demoralised.

Once the hospital returned to its normal complement of patients everyone managed to get some free time. We spent our days off in Alex – it was quite different; for one thing it was a busy port with ships coming and going all the time – big ships, little ships, Arab dhows and yachts. At the other end of the coast were the remains of the Pharos Lighthouse, one of the Seven Wonders of the World, and behind it one of the King of Egypt's palaces, all along the promenade were the beaches, many private, with spotless sand. The Cecil was the best hotel and there were good shops and patisseries, none to equal Pastroudis and a famous brothel called Mary's House (for officers only). Several British officers were killed there the night of the bombing and were listed as 'killed on active service', which I suppose was fair enough. Holed up in the harbour was part of the Vichy French fleet, there for the duration of the war. They were paid their normal wages and had nothing to do except keep their ships clean and in working order. They strutted about the town and there were endless fights between them and the Free French. Some of their crew tried to escape and join the Free French but it was not easy for them and, if caught, they were severely punished.

One officer – Roger Barbarot – did escape after two attempts. He was a very strong swimmer, which was just as well. At the first attempt he was pursued by a Vichy gunboat which ran him down and tried to drown him. He was captured and thrown into the hold; after several days of incarceration he succeeded in prising open the small porthole of his prison and, in the dark, managed to squirm out unseen to be rescued by an Arab fisherman in a dhow and put ashore. He made his way to the Free French HQ and joined the Foreign Legion, where he remained for several months. He then had a row with General Koenig and transferred to the French Marines – more navy than military – and remained with them until the end of the war. He served with great distinction and was the most decorated and famous officer in the Free French.

Buseilli was a nest of thieves. The fellahin were so poor that it was difficult not to feel sympathy towards them, but it was mixed with irritation when our stores were continually broken into. A trail of sugar led to a nearby village after one raid but the culprits were never caught. The Colonel decided that the only course of action was to increase our own guards and bring in better trained ones from the Brigade whose instructions were to fire first and ask questions afterwards. This certainly put a stop to the pilfering but not before one of our own men was shot when creeping in from a late assignment.

The Egyptians were the supreme masters of theft. Nothing was safe from them. Motor cars were particularly vulnerable. Drivers who sat in their cars for any length of time without getting out and taking a walk around them every ten minutes or so would discover, when they tried to drive away, that they no longer had any wheels. Another equally successful trick was for a small boy to make a sign at the back wheel of a vehicle; the driver would jump out thinking he had a flat tyre, and another urchin would be in at the off-side door collecting everything he could find.

In the heat of an Egyptian summer everyone drove with the windows open hoping to catch the slightest breeze. Unless drivers were particularly vigilant, packages would be snatched off the seats as they drove along the busy traffic-jammed streets. We soon learnt to lock everything in the boot of the car. While sleeping in his tent, Thibaux had everything stolen including the heavy tin trunk by his camp bed. Several people in our hospital woke up with the Egyptian sun beating down on them – their tents having disappeared while they were asleep inside. Some even claimed to have lost their camp beds while they were sleeping on them.

One evening, Solly Albert took a convoy of ambulances from Buseilli to Cairo containing convalescent wounded. They stopped for a few hours' sleep, but very soon Solly awoke with a start to discover an Arab about to remove the greatcoat he was sleeping in. The thief had already removed one of his arms from the sleeve, but was careless about the second one and Solly woke up in the nick of time.

The whole Hospital missed Lady Spears when she had to return to the Levant in November. We knew that she had a great deal of important work to do there as the wife of the British Minister to Syria and the Lebanon. Not only did she have to entertain the endless stream of officials and cabinet ministers who generally stayed at the Residence during their visits, but she also took a great interest in the Spears' missions and clinics which were dotted about the Levant.

Our Hospital was very dependant on her as well. We were such a multifarious collection of nationalities and creeds that there were bound to be tensions at times. Whenever the temperature of the Hospital rose to boiling point Lady Spears would be cabled and within twenty-four hours of her arrival she would have everything under her control. She would begin by interviewing the chief protagonists and, of course, the Colonel and the heads of different sections, giving them the impression that she had all the time in the world and understood their problems. The differences would be ironed out and smoothed over. Real trouble-makers were sent packing and once more the hospital would be working on oiled wheels. She had time for everyone and everything and accomplished more in twenty-four hours than anyone else I have ever known. Her brain worked like quicksilver and her conclusions and decisions were invariably right. She was afraid of no one and quite prepared to beard the Commander-in-Chief of the Eighth Army and did so on more than one occasion when her Hospital was threatened. Her prestige in the French Brigade was enormous and she was admired and esteemed by everyone.

Christmas 1942 was a cheerful time at the hospital after the success of El Alamein. We were still at Buseilli. There were not many wounded left, and most of them were up and about. There was much to celebrate. The Battle of El Alamein had been decisively won, and Rommel and his army were being pursued up the desert by the victorious Eighth Army. The Americans and the First British Army had landed successfully in North Africa, and the Free French Brigade re-equipped and re-trained and enlarged to a Division, was waiting impatiently to join in the chase.

We had time to explore the banks of the Nile between Buseilli and Rosetta and went for several walks through the fertile fields. Biddy and I made friends with some of the fellahin. Most of them owned a donkey which was more precious to them than their wife – they could always find another wife, but if they lost their beast of burden they could seldom afford to buy another. The Egyptian donkey was a beautiful animal, mostly white and twice the size of the little British ones. In spite of their value they were badly treated, carrying loads of twice their size and often ridden by two men at a time. The men rode their donkeys with their wives following them behind on foot. The donkeys nearly always suffered from deep saddle sores and other wounds; their feet were badly neglected and they were beaten continuously on their heads and quarters.

I persuaded the Colonel to help one family; the husband invited me into his shack where his wife was seriously ill after childbirth. The Colonel went to see her and told me she had puerperal fever and would probably die if she did not go into hospital. He could not risk treating her for, if she died, as she probably would, he would be held responsible for her death. She did die because her husband could not afford to send her to hospital. He was left with two small children and the baby, but he did have a donkey and I expect he quickly found another wife.

The one person not celebrating Christmas was me. I had developed jaundice and tried to cure myself with violent games of squash, tennis and hockey against the Australian hospital nearby. The treatment did not work and I changed colour to a brilliant shade of yellow. The Colonel confined me to bed for a week on a strict diet of rice and water and not much else. I was ordered not to drink alcohol for a year. It took a whole year for the yellow to fade from the palms of my hands and my eyeballs.

At the beginning of January I was sent off with Kit to spend ten days' sick leave as guests of Kostia and Domina Rodocanachi at Luxor in lower Egypt on the Nile; also with us as guests were Domino's niece, Helen Virsco, and an officer called Jocelyn Drew. We stayed in great comfort in the luxurious Winter Palace Hotel on the banks of the Nile and forgot all about the war. We rode, played tennis, and each morning crossed the Nile in a felucca.

We travelled by night train from Alexandria in comfortable sleepers and arrived early the following morning at Luxor station where we were met by taxis from the Winter Palace Hotel. We spent the first few days visiting the most important tombs and temples of Karnak, Thebes, Medinet Habu and Deir el Medinehand, and then travelled to the Valley of the Queens where the temple and tomb of Queen Hatshepsut is situated, some distance from Luxor. We were escorted by a very pleasant and interesting guide called Aboudi to the tomb of Tutankhamen, and shown his magnificent encased mummy after which we visited the tombs of Set and one of the numerous sons of Rameses III. I became fascinated by the history of the pharaohs, their religion, their gods and their daily lives and bought all the books I could find on the subject. Some of the tombs we visited were of the pharaohs' officials, and depicted in brilliant colours scenes from their daily lives intermingled with birds, fish and animals. In the tombs of the kings and queens and princes and princesses, the pictures showed them being introduced to their various gods.

There were no tourists; we had the best guides to ourselves and were permitted to visit several tombs forbidden to the public. Aboudi gave me a piece of highly decorated mosaic from one of the tombs. When I showed it to Biddy on my return she gave a scream of horror, said it was unlucky and made me throw it into the Mediterranean – something I have regretted ever since.

Near Assouan we visited an excavation of newly discovered tombs which was being directed by a French archaeologist. He was completely ignorant of the war and cared less; his whole life was wrapped up in Egyptology and the search for a tomb which had not been plundered. The only one discovered to date is that of Tutankhamen.

We were driven to Thebes or to the Valley of the Kings and Queens in antique taxis, tyres patched with pieces of rags, which were continuously boiling over or breaking down. After a few days we changed to a more reliable mode of transport – the magnificent Egyptian white donkey, twice the size of the European and very sure footed and strong.

We visited the Cataracts of Assouan and inspected the series of locks and dams controlling the flow water in the Nile. We sailed to Kitchener's Island and Elephant Island, an island belonging to an Egyptian princess, full of orange and lemon trees and exotic flowers. All in all, we lived the life of rich tourists at the Rodocanachis' expense instead of being drivers in a hospital unit. I enjoyed it very much indeed and felt much better as well. I celebrated my birthday there with a large cake provided by the hotel.

When Kit and I returned to the hospital on 19 January 1943 we learnt that we were moving with the Division to Tobruk on 22 January. After living the life of the idle rich I was quickly brought back to reality. The cars all had to be serviced, checked and packed. The patients were all evacuated from the hospital wards which were then packed up and loaded on to the trucks. We left at 7.30am led by Michael Rowntree in his biscuit tin of a van, and joined the divisional convoy on the road to Alexandria. Every vehicle in our convoy was loaded to capacity and carried, as well as the hospital and our own equipment, a curious collection of livestock including dogs, cats, pigeons and chickens.

As we were seven drivers with only five staff cars, we took over two of the water buggies and I drove one of them on this first day. Amazingly for Egypt, where the average rainfall is practically nil, it was pouring with rain when we set off and several of the trucks refused to start so it was quite a business getting the convoy off in time and in one piece. In fact, my water buggy lived up to its name. The cabin had neither roof nor windscreen, so the rain drove into my face, which made if difficult to see, and I was soon drenched to the skin and very cold.

We halted just before Alexandria for a check count of vehicles and then drove to Amarya to refuel. The desert on this part of the journey was refreshingly green with fig and olive tree plantations on either side of the road, the surface of which was appalling: what the French call *bombe* – corrugated, and full of pot and bomb holes. At Amarya, due to muddled orders, we lost half the convoy. It had been mistakenly diverted and did not catch us up again until we reached Bourg el Arab.

We saw the first signs of the Battle of El Alamein soon after leaving Bourg el Arab. The débris of war was to become an all-too-familiar sight and always the same – burnt out trucks, tanks and planes, tank tracks, ammunition boxes, petrol cans, boots, tin hats, pieces of uniform, tyres. And paper, paper everywhere – newspaper, lavatory paper, writing paper, order sheets, maps, letters – all blowing about in the wind, desolated and deserted. There were minefields too. Tangles of barbed wire enclosed some of them. The British marked theirs with the names of rivers and the way through them with the names of London gates, Stanhope Gate, Hyde Park Gate, and so on. The Germans, on the other hand, marked theirs all the same, a skull and crossbones with *Achtung Minen* (Beware Mines) underneath. Soldiers' graves were dotted around, some with wooden crosses with the soldier's name inscribed in ink. The German crosses had a swastika outlined in black. Many graves had no crosses, only a tin hat on a bayonet with an identity disc attached.

The Italians were reported to have put booby traps around their dead and when the RASC arrived to bury them they were blown up. After several deaths and injuries they refused to bury any more and the Italian prisoners were made to bury their own dead.

In the desert are soldiers' graves.
Where the jackal cries
And the gazelle roams
By the shores of the sea.
It is lonely in the desert.

They are alone now.
Lying where their tanks blazed
And machine-guns spattered
And shrapnel penetrated
Into their soft flesh.

And the men who buried them
Put up wooden crosses,
Writing their names in pencil
Or on paper in a bottle,
So that they would not be forgotten.
But there are some with no names
Only their rifles or tin hats
Which are no identification.
It is quiet in the desert.

Perhaps when this war is over
A committee or trust
Will build a cemetery
And gather up the crosses
And the bottles and rifles.

But I think it would be kinder
To leave them to their loneliness
With only the jackals' call
And the sea's moan.
For there is peace in the desert.

R H-E

The Italians were also accused of tying dogs to mines which exploded when the dogs were released. They seemed to put booby traps wherever they could, in all bombed and empty buildings, also scattering anti-personnel bombs in the form of thermos flasks and fountain pens. We were forbidden to pick up any suspicious-looking object.

We passed one large enemy airfield which was strewn with wrecked planes, mostly Italian. I counted over thirty as we drove past and there were many more. In places the road had completely disappeared and we were diverted across sand which had been turned into a quagmire by the rain. Vehicles kept getting stuck and had to be pulled or dug out by our maintenance crew who always followed behind at the end of the convoy to help anyone who had fallen by the wayside. They always had a hard day's work. Our brand-new operating theatre truck, of which we were so proud and which had been a present to us from our friends the Rodocanachis in Alexandria, was the worst offender and kept breaking down as well as getting stuck in the mud. We finally reached Daaba, our leaguer for the night. We filled up with petrol before doing anything else. There were puddles and mud everywhere but we were lucky enough to be next door to the NAAFI where we were given a hot meal of bacon and eggs. Iris and I, who drove the buggies, were soaked to the skin and shivering with cold, so we were lent a tent for the night by the NAAFI padre. He also dried our shirts and trousers. So at least we were protected from the rain, even though the ground below was rather damp. Everyone else had to sleep in their cars or trucks.

On 23 January we set off at 7.30am again with most of our vehicles roadworthy. I had been switched to driving a staff car and had as passengers Père Boileau and Colonel Simonitch – a Polish doctor attached to the hospital for a short while. We drove through Fuka and Garola, names on a board with a few army huts and wooden posts scattered around, nothing to indicate that they were worthy of a name on a map. We thought they were probably Bedouin wells in the days before the war.

The road gradually became less monotonous with bends and gradients and in the distance we could see small hills leading down to the sea, with empty white beaches and the iridescent blue of the Mediterranean. The rain had stopped. We arrived at the Egyptian watering town of Mersa Matruh. Before the war rich Egyptians and the foreign colony of Egypt had villas here where they spent their weekends. Italian divers lived here as well, diving for the best sponges in the world. When we arrived, we found the town had been shelled and bombed by each advancing and retreating army and there was little left standing amongst the ruins. The shell of a mosque, a church, the walls of a hotel, the rubble of the governor's house, the remains of shops and houses were all deserted now and probably mined. Here we caught up with a heavy army convoy moving very slowly which we were able to pass. Mike Rowntree decided to stop at a wayside NAAFI and let the convoy get well ahead of us. The débris of war again was everywhere and we were reminded not to touch anything and be careful where we walked as there were booby traps and anti-personnel mines lying around.

We halted for the night on the outskirts of Sidi Barrani, which we could see nothing of as it was dark when we arrived. Tired from our long drive we quickly went to sleep, either beside our cars or inside them.

The final day of our convoy drive began, as usual, at 7.30am. A few vehicles had dropped out, including Rosie Forbes and Barbara Graham in their staff car. The car had a broken chassis but they expected to have this repaired in time to catch us up before we arrived at Tobruk. I was back driving a water buggy again. Dry and crisp, the morning was perfect with early sun. We drove through Sidi Barrani, the buildings glaring white in the dawn. Only when we drew nearer did we realise that once again all the buildings were empty shells and in ruins. A few Arabs were wandering around offering 'eggies' for sale or bartering for cigarettes. The desert road straightened out after Sidi Barrani and the colour of the sand changed from pale yellow to brick red. Tank traps across the road every few miles and an increased amount of traffic in both directions slowed down our progress considerably. Minefields ran along each side of the road with small clearances for British, German and Italian cemeteries. Everywhere there were wrecked tanks and lorries.

Through Buq Buq – yet another name on a board at the side of the road – and on to Sollum, which is sited in the most magnificent position overlooking the sea which forms a bay around it. There was not a building left in the lower town but above the pass and through the escarpment in the upper town there were a few Egyptian forts with only roof and windows missing. We climbed up Sollum pass (christened 'Hell Fire Pass' by the British) along a wide road which winds its way up the precipitous cliff overhanging the sea – a hard test for any vehicle and, at the slow speed of the convoy, most of our trucks and all our staff cars were boiling over by the time we reached the top. Soon after Sollum we approached and passed the Egyptian–Libyan frontier, Fort Capuzzu, the Italian border fortress where the remains of a deep barbed-wire fence reinforced with concrete stretched as far as we could see into the desert. We bypassed Bardia, the first Italian town. There were many more Arabs here, with herds of camels which wandered around the deserted barracks. We passed Gambut, yet another name on a board, and soon afterwards were halted at one of the Free French camps for further instructions. Here we were made to disperse our vehicles in case of air attacks, which were frequent and always frightening. Stukas would come out of nowhere and machine gun any vehicle they could find. Our staff cars were prime targets; they probably thought that there was a general on board. We would either stop the car and hurl ourselves into the roadside ditch, if there was one (which was not very often), or drive at speed in circles across the desert – if it was not mined!

As soon as we received our instructions we moved on and had two more halts before our destination, a wadi, some six miles from Tobruk and a few miles from the sea. It was too dark to see much and we got out our bedding and dossed down. In all we had completed 750 kilometres in three days driving, with the maximum speed of the slowest vehicle about 20 miles per hour.

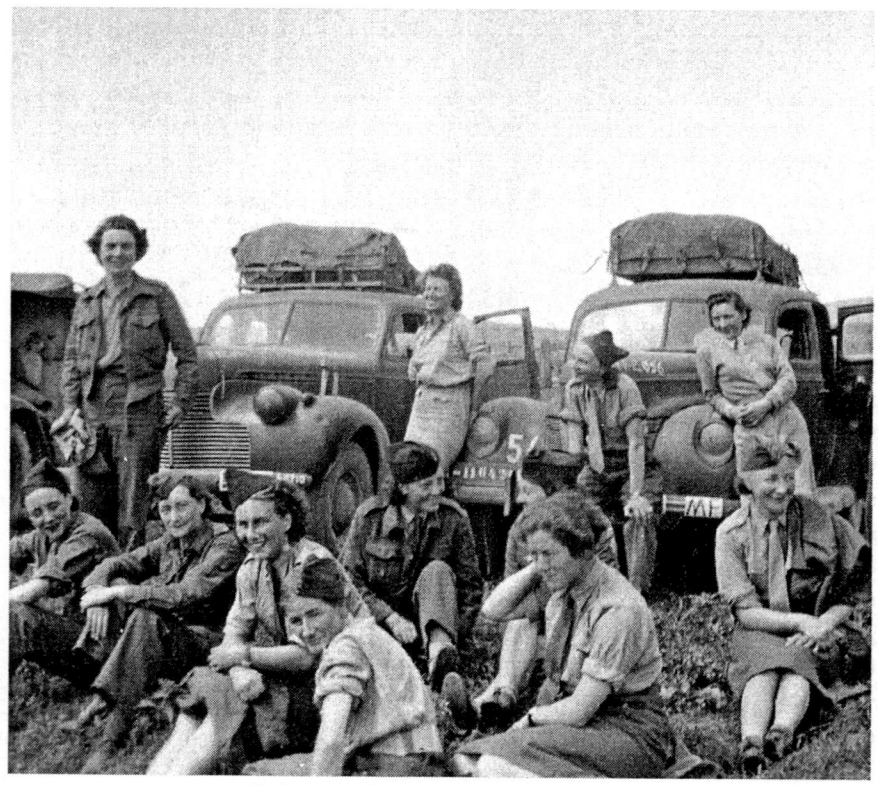

Drivers and nurses at a convoy stop.

3

LIFE IN THE DESERT

When we inspected our site in daylight we were delighted to discover that we were perched on top of the wadi. We set up our tented hospital and operating theatre, ordnance, workshops, mess tents and kitchen sited on flat ground. The trucks were garaged at one side of the complex and our staff cars were lined up on a piece of ground between a series of ravines. Our own tents were sited on the side of another wadi, nearer to and overlooking the sea. The FAU put up all the tents with their usual speed and efficiency and in no time at all the hospital was in working order and ready to receive patients.

Here we settled down for almost three months, the longest time we ever spent in one place. By the end of our sojourn our living quarters looked more like a gypsy encampment than a military hospital. Several of us had built our own dwellings: Rose, for instance, had scraped together a collection of empty petrol cans, piled them one on top of the other and roofed them with a piece of tarpaulin. Every time it rained the roof collapsed and when the wind blew the tarpaulin went with it. However, she always succeeded in finding it. Jean Williams had married Pat Barr, a member of the FAU, before we left Buseilli and they built themselves a very superior hut out of orange boxes and scrap which they had found in an old Italian army dump. Their house boasted a front door, a window and a roof of corrugated iron. They even carved a small garden out of the sand and planted it with flowers they dug out of the desert. Barbara originally pitched her tent in a very picturesque spot overlooking the sea. Unfortunately it was in the path of a dried up stream and, when it rained more heavily than usual one night, all her belongings floated out of her tent and down the stream to the sea. She and her camp bed were washed against one of the tent poles which woke her up before she also floated away to the sea. Biddy, Iris, Jocelyn and myself shared a bell tent where we just had room for an orange box and our tin trunks between each bed. We bought straw mats from the Arabs to put on the ground between the beds, which helped to keep the sand out of our belongings. We hung our great-coats and mackintoshes from the hooks which held the tent together, and draped the uniform we wore each day on strings, which we stretched from pole to pole and which were always collapsing.

The rainy season in Tobruk lasted about three weeks and during this time flowers sprang out of nowhere and everywhere. The desert became a veritable 'Garden of Eden', such a variety which put even the English show gardens in competition. Jocelyn had a field day and spent all her off duty collecting, identifying and painting all she could find. I collected twenty different species for her from one spot. Not only were there annuals that one might expect but shrubs like broom and lavinia. Growing in great confusion were poppies, rock roses, thrift, saxifrage, many different coloured daisies, asters and cacti and many more – surprisingly lupins, delphiniums, irises and dozens of others. All they required was water. How could they shoot up in such a short time, and what happened to them when the rain ceased and everywhere became unbearably hot? Did they spring from seeds or were there roots deep down in the sand? It really was a miracle. With the flowers came the birds – sand grouse, pipits, larks, swallows and, of course, sparrows. Sometimes we saw a gazelle in the distance. Tortoises were common; we saw the odd snake, and less welcome scorpion. It was said that only scorpions of the same size would mate; if one was larger it would sting the other to death. Mergier collected them to see if it was true but never succeeded in keeping a pair alive.

We had to be careful about scorpions, they liked to get into empty shoes or flea-bags or clothes lying around. The yellow ones had a painful sting but the black ones were really dangerous. Luckily for us the black ones were very rare. Rosie was stung by a yellow one when she was driving along with me. She started wriggling about saying something was stinging her so we stopped and she found a scorpion up one of her trouser legs.

In Egypt we encountered everything that bit or stung. In Cairo the gharries, taxis, the arms of the wicker chairs on the verandas at Shepheard's Hotel and the seats at the open air cinemas were all infested with bugs which gave a nasty bite. The mosquitoes were malarial so we had to take one atebrin a day which had nasty side effects. We thought that the fleas at Tobruk might have been left behind by the Italians who had a camp nearby before they were captured. Last, but not least, were the flies who arrived in such hordes that it was difficult to take a mouthful of food without swallowing half a dozen flies as well.

Water was always a scarce commodity in the desert. We were given a personal allowance of two gallons a week, which included drinking water apart from that which was provided in the mess. Whenever we complained we were told how privileged we were to be part of a hospital as the ration for each soldier in the Eighth Army was only one gallon a week. Everyone had their own system of eking out their ration and many were the discussions and inventions. Petrol, unlike water, was in plentiful supply and it was not long before we were washing our battle dress and skirts in petrol. Paraffin was also plentiful and we washed our hair in this. Once the hair was dry it didn't smell but we had to be careful not to rub it into the scalp as it burnt the skin. Curiously it gave our hair a beautiful shine and did not seem to do it any harm. Even with these economies the water still had a long way to go, giving rise to further discussions – did you wash your face or your teeth first? What about the rest of your body? Your underclothes and shirts? Most people could not wash these in petrol or paraffin because they were liable to cause a rash.

The water at Tobruk was unbelievable – talk to anyone who has drunk it and watch the expression on their face. Each retreating army had polluted the wells; dead donkeys, corpses, and anything else was chucked in so that the water, which still flowed and was the army's only source, had to be highly chlorinated for safety's sake. Brackish and salty, it had a bouquet of its own (whisky, tea or coffee could not disguise it) but no one died from drinking it and we were thirsty enough to have to.

We were lucky in that we possessed four water buggies and these we sent twice weekly to Derna to collect 'sweet water' for the hospital and mess. Even that was highly chlorinated and flat but a great improvement on the water of Tobruk. Of all the things we did without in the desert, a glass of sparkling cold water was what we missed most. Whenever it rained, as it did frequently the first month we were in Tobruk, we would rush out and put buckets, tins, basins and anything that held water, under the flaps of our tents to catch the precious drops. This we saved for drinking and, if there was any left over, for washing our hair, bodies and clothes.

Some of the rain storms were very unpleasant. The wind usually blew strongly at the same time and the combination of wind and rain pulled and loosened the tent pegs out of the wet sand. We had a continuous fight to prevent the tents from collapsing. Tent poles would sway drunkenly, there would be an ominous crack, a tearing of the guy ropes and 'flop' – down would come the tent on our heads. It was no joke in the middle of the night with driving rain outside, in pitch darkness with everything soaking – wet beds, clothes, ourselves, the lot. Often our precious matches were soaked as well and it was impossible to find or light the one hurricane lamp which had been hanging on a tent rope. Someone always came to our aid and luckily these storms did not last many hours. Soon the sun would shine again and everything could be brought out to dry. The rain turned the sand into a sticky glue which clung as tenaciously as the heaviest clay but was much softer. Vehicles were bogged down below their axles and tracks became impassable. When the ruts made by the churning trucks dried out they did even more damage to the low undercarriages of our cars than the mud did to their transmissions.

All over the desert soldiers used petrol to brew up over their desert fires. The method was simplicity itself. Cut the top off a square British petrol can and fill it three-quarters full of sand. Pour petrol on to it , let it soak in, and throw a lighted match from a safe distance. The fire burnt merrily for long enough to boil a kettle, or cook an egg or a tin of bully beef. We received several terrible burn cases; soldiers who had tried to revive dying fires by throwing more petrol on – whereupon the flames jumped back to the can, which exploded.

An easy way to make drinking glasses was to fill a whisky or beer bottle three-quarters full of engine oil and plunge a red-hot bayonet into it. The glass would crack and break off at the height of the oil; the rim could then be smoothed ready for use.

It was bitterly cold in our wadi for the first few weeks and the hospital quickly filled up with accident and medical cases. A few days after our arrival I was asked to go on night duty as several sisters were on leave. The hospital wards were freezing. Slippery duckboards ran down the middle of the tents, and sacking was put by each bed in an attempt to soak up some of the damp. The patients complained incessantly as they pulled their blankets over their heads and I sat, huddled over the one and only paraffin stove, wearing my greatcoat, with a blanket over my shoulders and a hot water bottle on my knees. The cold penetrated the warmest clothes although the temperature never fell below freezing. The damp crept into everything and we had no way of drying anything except in the sun. The wind blew the double flaps of the tents together and, wherever they touched, water leaked through and drips of water fell on to beds, patients and dressings. Fleas added to the general misery; huge and rapacious, they multiplied in the humidity. Flit and DDT made no impression on them whatsoever. Some people were immune to their bites but not me; I could feel them crawling all over my body and biting me. However many times I stripped off my clothes, deloused myself and covered my body with DDT, I never got rid of them and I was covered in so many bites that I looked as if I had chicken pox. I even put the feet of my camp bed in empty cigarette tins filled with paraffin but nothing helped until the hot weather returned and they disappeared. What was so annoying was that my orderly, Pat Barr, never got bitten at all and used to laugh at me in my misery.

Very often one could see a khamseen (sand storm) approaching like a wall of yellow, blotting out everything behind it. One soldier wrote home: 'They say there is 2,000 miles of sand in the Western desert – 1,000 miles has just blown over me'. The Bedouin say that a khamseen blows for one, three or seven days and by the seventh men go mad. I could well believe it. The desert is a strange place and no man is indifferent to it; he either loves it or hates it. There were so many contrasts and extremes, heat and cold, drought and floods, hot winds, cold winds and mostly no wind at all. Space and freedom, loneliness and silence. So much is unexpected: the birds singing, gazelle, tortoises and scorpions appearing from nowhere. Here one sees the most beautiful sunrises and sunsets in the world. A luminosity quite unique changes the colour of the yellow and white sand to rosy hues, sending back shadows which are caught and reflected by the sky. The midday sun, when a haze of heat shimmers and dances and produces strange fantasies, provides mirages of green oases, caravans of camels and ships at sea, miles out in the desert.

The town of Tobruk was about eight miles from our wadi, built on a hill overlooking the harbour. Before the war singled it out as a key position, it must have been a pleasant port. It was in ruins by the time we reached it in January 1943; not a single building was left intact. Most of the hospital was rubble, the church was a shell. Navy House and the rows of small white-washed houses, built in the Italian colonial style, were nearly all totally demolished. When we arrived we found that, apart from the military had taken charge of the harbour which was full of wrecks. Rumour had it that there were over 200 lying there and, indeed, they were so thickly packed that not even a rowing boat could pass between them or a sprat swim through. No ship could get in or out until the Navy made a channel.

Around the outskirts of Tobruk were war cemeteries, one for each nationality who had fought in the desert. Everywhere there was the wreckage of war. There were minefields, often unmarked, and the wandering Senussi and their camels were continually getting blown up and many of the casualties were brought to our Hospital.

Much to our relief our Division was being rested, refitted and retrained after the losses of men and material at El Alamein. The hospital fell into an easy routine where most of our patients were medical cases with just the odd accident case and surgical operation.

We spent many hours exploring the neighbouring wadis and the surrounding desert for the wrecked and abandoned Fords to pick to pieces for any spare parts that would come in useful for our own cars. During our foraging we came across quite a few things to improve the comfort of our tents, such as ammunition boxes, bayonets and German water bottles, which were vastly superior to the British ones.

A few weeks after we had settled down at Tobruk, Kit's boxer bitch Olga – who had travelled with us in convoy with her two remaining puppies which Kit had promised to officers in the Queen's Bays – began behaving very strangely. She took a violent dislike to one of her puppies, refused her food and ate dirt instead. She became generally hysterical and excitable, quite out of character as she was normally a very placid and gentle dog. The Colonel examined her and said she was almost certainly suffering from milk fever as her other six puppies had been left behind in Cairo and there had been no time to wean them properly. Unfortunately, we had the nasty feeling that she might have rabies. A few days later she had become very much worse, unable to swallow and dribbling saliva continuously. The Colonel genially gave Kit permission to take her to the Pasteur Institute at Alexandria for examination. He still insisted that she had not got rabies. He claimed to have seen many cases of the disease and was positive that she was not showing any of the symptoms.

We had a terrible time getting Olga into the back of the car without being bitten. Her eyes were bright red; she could hardly stand up and had diarrhoea. We finally managed to lift her in and tie her on to the back seat with ropes and leads, so that she could not jump over on to the front seat of the car. Kit and Biddy set off, Kit driving and Biddy facing Olga with a loaded revolver and gloves ready to shoot her if she broke loose and attacked them. They had a nightmare journey. Olga managed to get loose twice and tore and bit all the upholstery in the back of the car to ribbons. They succeeded in getting her tied up each time she broke loose as they had promised the Colonel to get her down to Alexandria alive and not to shoot her, except in desperation. The party eventually arrived in Alexandria at midnight and went directly to the Pasteur Institute where they left the dog. The following morning they learnt that she had died and that the clinical examination pointed strongly to rabies.

We, in the meantime, had collected hurdles from Bir Hakim and made a kennel for the puppies to keep them in some sort of quarantine until we received news from Alexandria. Later both puppies were destroyed.

Lady Spears and Mrs Richard Casey, wife of the Australian Minister of State in Cairo, flew in to visit the hospital the day after Kit and Biddy left. We did our best to make them as comfortable as possible. The signal from Alexandria was delivered the evening of their arrival 'Suspected rabies – all contacts report to the Pasteur Clinic in Cairo immediately'. Captain Thibaux, Barbara Graham and I had all helped to look after Olga and her puppies and had been bitten or licked by her, as had Iris and Aimee who were away on leave. We thought that they were in Cyprus or Crete but no one really knew. GHQ Cairo eventually ran them to ground and arranged that they should immediately be sent to Cairo for treatment.

Thibaux, Barbara and I left the following morning in a Wellington bomber which had been diverted from its flight from London to Cairo to pick us up at El Adem airfield – 'three interesting cases'. We had quite a long wait at the airfield and amused ourselves by running around the field barking at each other. The officer in charge was quite worried; he really thought we were rabid. I played the same trick some time later in Cairo on a Madame D'Assonville who had insisted on censoring our letters on the *Pasteur*. I met her on the way back from the Pasteur clinic one morning in the Mohammed Ali Street. She grasped my hand and I gave a bark and a growl and explained why I was in Cairo. She dropped my hand like a hot brick and shot across the street – and was nearly run over by a tram.

The Wellington bomber was not built to carry passengers, so we were all cramped into the middle gun turret. The plane flew at only 18,000 feet and we had a wonderful view. The sea was so blue that day that I was reminded of D H Lawrence's poem: 'This sea will never die, neither will it ever grow old nor cease to be blue'. Just before El Alamein we branched off right-handed over the desert and had a plane's eye view of the battle area – every wheel track, every dug-out, pup hole and gun site, every bomb crater and shell hole clearly visible.

While we three were wending our way down to Cairo, Biddy and Kit had returned to the hospital in Tobruk with enough anti-rabies serum for all of us. The Colonel, however, said that it was useless as it had to be kept at a continuous temperature of just below freezing point and it had already been spoilt during the journey. So, in spite of having driven through the night with no sleep, they were put on the next plane back to Cairo and joined us there the following day.

The anti-rabies treatment was very unpleasant – a daily injection of 10ccs for fifteen days from a very long (and not always sharp) needle into the stomach. The first few were not too bad but after the sixth or seventh the whole abdominal area became swollen and tender and most of us developed a body rash as well. We were told not to drink any alcohol or to have a hot bath – a luxury after the waterless desert was too much to forego and we needed a sun-down tipple to keep us going.

During the time we were enduring our daily anti-rabies injections, I furthered my study of ancient Egypt by visiting the pyramids of Sakara and Memphis and the surrounding tombs. These were much earlier than the tombs of Karnak; the decorations on their walls were carved in relief and not painted, they were more stylised but gave the same pictures of the daily life of their inhabitants.

We set off every morning at nine for the Pasteur clinic and joined a long queue – never fewer than fifty – of people of all ages from small babies to old men. We were told by Russell Pasha, Barbara's uncle, that many Egyptians believed that the anti-rabies treatment cured them of opium addiction and that probably half the men having injections were not rabies contacts at all. They must have been desperate to voluntarily undergo such a disagreeable cure.

By the time we had completed our fifteen days' treatment we had learnt a great deal about rabies. We had been on conducted tours round the laboratories and also the hospital wards, where two

Egyptians were dying of the disease. We were told that we could still develop the disease up to two years after the treatment, which was a cheerful thought.

One day, while we were living at Tobruk, Kit and I were returning from some mission in the desert a long way from the only road which followed the coast line. We were driving on a compass bearing when we suddenly came across a signpost saying *Achtung Minen* and realised that we were in the middle of a minefield. Kit was driving in La Belle Marguerite and came to an abrupt halt. I realised that it was entirely my fault – although we had a compass, which I was holding, I had insisted that we were too far over on the right – which was the opposite to the truth. We looked at each other in dismay. 'Well,' said Kit, 'while we are still alive and can enjoy it let's have a tot of whisky to calm our nerves'. 'Why not?' I said. 'It may well be our last'. We both had a good swig at the bottle then I said: 'There's only one thing to do; I will get out and walk behind you guiding you while you reverse on your tracks'. All went well, we had another swig and then found our way back to the hospital. Needless to say, we never told anyone as we were not very proud of ourselves and would have got no sympathy.

Lady Spears and Mrs Casey had left by the time I returned to the unit. The Hospital was less than half full. We, the drivers, spent our days driving and maintaining our cars. Two drivers were always on duty and if the rest were not needed they were more or less free to do what they liked.

There were many parties at this time with the various regiments of the Division. General de Larminat and General Koenig and other top brass invited us to meals at the HQs. The SAS and the Long Range Desert Group often used us as halfway house of their way to and from their missions behind the enemy lines, as did our friends in the Eighth Army. It was a very happy time and everyone was given leave – except the rabid ones.

4

THE LONGEST CONVOY DRIVE

The First Division of the Free French was concentrated between Tobruk and Bardia where it was being re-grouped by General de Larminat for retraining with new equipment. The regiments of the division, to which new recruits arrived in a steady stream, were to remain the same until the end of the war. It was made up of three brigades. The first consisted of the 13th Demi-brigade of the Foreign Legion and the 22nd North African Battalion. The Second brigade was made up of the 3rd, 4th, 5th and 11th Battalions of de Marche – all African – while the Third brigade consisted of the 21st and 24th Battalion de Marche and the Battalion de Marine et Pacifique. Completing the division was the Artillerie, the First regiment of the Fusiliers Marins (the French equivalent of the Royal Marines – mostly naval officers and personnel who had no ship to serve in and so were 'land sailors'), le Génie (sappers), le Train, l'Intendence, Transmissions, Réparations, la Circulation Routière, the Ambulance Chirurgicale and our group – the Hadfield–Spears Hospital.

From June 1942 until May 1943 Headquarters was commanded by General Legentilhomme. In May 1943 General Koenig commanded briefly until July, followed by de Larminat from December 1943 to April 1944. General Brosset then took over until 20 November 1944 when he was tragically killed. From then until the end of the war General Garbay was in command.

The officers and men were a varied and diverse collection. Many of them had been condemned to death by the Vichy government and a few of these, like General de Larminat and General Koenig, had a price on their heads. To join de Gaulle and the Free French many of them had travelled far, some from France, through Spain, Switzerland or Portugal. Others had arrived from the Congo, Madagascar, French North Africa or, like General Catroux, from Indo-China. A few, such as René Millet – my future husband – first escaped from a German prisoner of war camp at the beginning of 1941 to Russia, where they were immediately imprisoned in a series of concentration camps and endured the rigours of being Russian political prisoners, before being rescued by the British Navy in August 1941 and arriving with us in 1942.

The story of René's escape from a PoW camp in Germany to Russia and his release from there is worth telling. He was taken prisoner with the rest of his regiment when France was overrun by the

Germans and capitulated. He was then sent to an officers' PoW camp in Pomerania and immediately started planning his escape. Five of them decided to attempt together, Charles de Pomplonne, Meyer (nicknamed the 'jockey' because he was so small), a Pole called Mittelle who became well-known after the war for his cartoons, René, and a fifth who was picked up by the Germans when they reached a railway station. They were helped by Jean Marin who, after the war, became Manager of the Plaza Athenée Hotel in Paris. He supplied them with false documents, civilian clothes and maps.

The elderly German officer in charge of the PoW camp had fought in the 1914 war. René announced to him that he was going to escape the following day. The German roared with laughter and said: 'You Frenchmen with your sense of humour. I assure you, you will not escape. I was a prisoner with the British in the last war and I never succeeded.' True to his word René and his companions left punctually at midday. They bluffed the guards with false passes describing them as Polish workmen who were working in the prison. All went well until they reached the station at Konigsberg where they lost their fifth companion. They left the train somewhere on the Friedland Plateau and walked all night, not very sure where they were. At daybreak they reached a swollen river full of ice-floes. René, being the only strong swimmer, had to cross the river three times to ferry his companions across. He suffered frostbite in one of his ears for the rest of his life and only just escaped frostbitten feet as well. He chums spent an hour massaging his feet and lent him their dry socks.

The river was the boundary between Germany and Russia and they had not walked many yards before they were arrested by Russian guards. Then their troubles really began. They were thrown into prison as political spies, the worst category of prisoners in Russia. This was in spite of the fact that Germany had invaded Russia, and they kept repeating that they were French officers who had escaped from Germany to join the Free French. They were moved from prison to prison, beaten, starved and abused. Luckily for them there were also British prisoners who had escaped from Germany. Their fate had become known to MacFarlan, the British Military Attaché in Moscow, who advised the British government not to send the Russians any much-needed arms until they coughed up their British prisoners. The Russians, after repeatedly denying that they had any British prisoners, eventually released them. They told MacFarlan that there were some fifty French PoWs also held by the Russians; among them Captain Bilotte, son of a French General, who happened to be a friend of MacFarlan's. At first the Russians denied having any French prisoners but they did finally release them.

René said that the Russians had an extraordinary mentality and that they genuinely believed the French wanted to remain in Russia. They were heavily guarded all the way from their prison to the quayside where they embarked on a British warship, which was on its way to Spitzbergen with a flotilla of ships carrying British and Canadian troops to destroy the coal mining installations and refineries and heavy water factory before they reached Germany.

René weighed only seven stone when he was released and the others were in a similar state. He told me that the sailors helping them on board were in tears when they saw their condition. He said that after they had been washed, deloused, fed and medically inspected they were each given a uniform and a responsible job to do. He admitted that they were hardly capable but they felt their morale return and they felt like human beings again. René said this, more than anything else, restored them and that only the British Navy would have thought of such a thing.

When the four finally reached England they all joined up with the Free French. Pomplonne joined de Gaulle's HQ as the diplomat he was, René to the French Navy and then the FM and our Division, just after the battle of El Alamein.

With one or two exceptions the officers in the Division were French, while the ranks were of every nationality, colour and creed. The majority had done no more training than their national service and many not even that. They came from all walks of life: fishermen, farmers, diplomats, gangsters, doctors, priests, businessmen, labourers and peasants – all united under the Croix de Lorraine and ready and willing to lay down their lives for France.

I met René Millet for the first time in Tobruk. He later claimed that his truck had got stuck in the sand outside the Hospital and he was wandering around looking for help when he saw a pair of legs sticking out from beneath a car. Apparently, when he got no reply to his appeals for help, he leaned down and pulled the legs and, to his amazement, he found they belonged to a girl, filthy dirty, covered in grease and oil, who let fly a stream of oaths in broken Tirailleuse French at him. He swore it was me and that I eventually calmed down and invited him to our tent for a drink while someone dug out his truck. It must have been the whisky which made him decide that I was worth cultivating, for a few days later he invited Rosie and me to a dinner party at Gambut.

We dressed for the dinner, putting on our best uniform, clean shirt with immaculately tied tie, and polished Sam Browne belt. René, who.

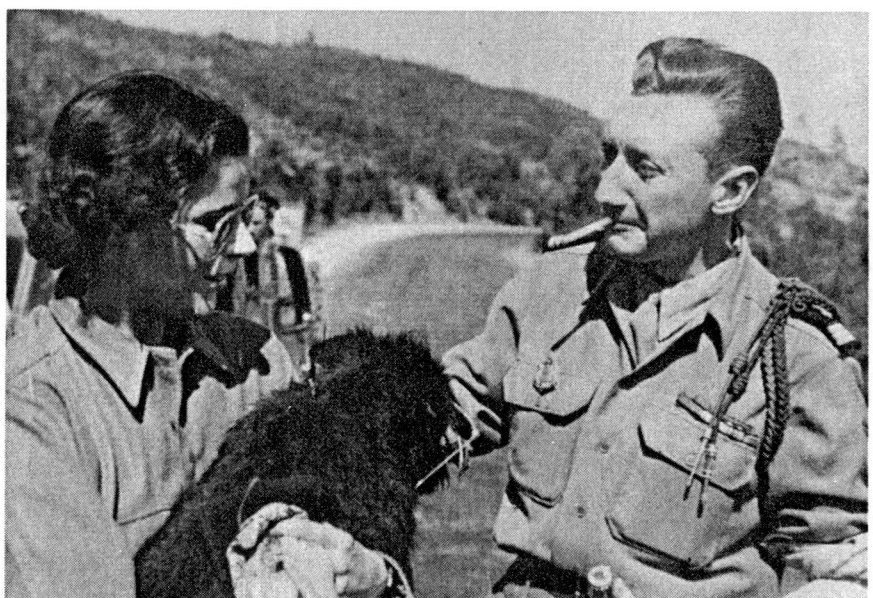

Rosie, Bazooka and René.

arrived with his best friend and fellow officer Philippe le Bourgeoise, said he could not believe the transformation. They had arrived with two trucks and drivers to collect us. I went with René, who drove like a bat out of hell and frightened me so much that I firmly resolved that nothing was going to make me drive with him again. We missed some vehicles by inches and scraped past others, bending a mudguard and wing. Finally, having weaved in and out of shell holes and skidded on and off the road, we turned down a track which led to the sea.

There, waiting for us, were more of his fellow officers and a gramophone playing South Sea Island tunes. Lanterns and torches were arranged in a semi-circle around a feast laid out on the beach. It was quite a party and the menu was no mean achievement in the middle of the desert in war time.

GAMBUT PALM BEACH   7.IV.43
Hors d'Œuvres à la Bougainville
Poulet Tahiti
Macédoine des Légumes
Pommes Sauteés
Salade Kerguelen
Beignets Brestoises
Choix de Fruits des Iles
Rack, Tafia, Bière

The Poulet Tahiti was a bit tough – it had probably been stolen from the Arabs and chased all the way from Tobruk to Gambut. However, it was the best dinner we had eaten in the desert. At the end of the evening I was so anxious not to drive back with René that I climbed into Philippe's truck and asked him to drive me back, leaving Rosie to return with René. Apparently one of the hurricane lamps had caught fire in their truck and they had great difficulty putting it out before the truck blew up. They were furious with us for not waiting and didn't forgive us for a long time.

The dinner was a particular treat because our desert army rations were so monotonous and uninspiring. Our diet consisted of enormous loaves of bread, at least a week old and hard as a brick, thick biscuits which looked like dog biscuits, porridge, apricot jam (made mostly of turnip), marmalade, particularly disgusting pilchards in tomato sauce, the occasional tin of spam and the staple bully beef, which was always edible. Our Syrian cook, when he was not a patient in the VD ward, did the best he could and succeeded in producing an amazing variety of stews and fries with the bully beef. Sometimes we were lucky and drew a tin of apricots or pineapple with the rations, and from time to time Père Boileau (our Messing Officer) bought a tough chicken and pigeon-sized eggs from the Arabs. The eggs were usually stale and sometimes bad. A treat was tunny fish, which tasted more like meat than fish. We also had dates as dessert which sometimes caused the gripes but were welcome all the same. We never saw a fresh vegetable, or any other fruit than dates.

The drawback to this diet was not so much its lack of variety but lack of vitamins. Everyone suffered to a greater or lesser degree from vitamin deficiency which manifested itself as desert sores. A knock or a cut, or even a flea or mosquito bite on legs and arms, often refused to heal and became infected with a fungus which bit deeper and deeper into the flesh until it reached the bone. Many treatments were tried and failed. The Colonel finally discovered the best way was to slap on elastoplast and leave it there until it fell off of its own accord. This seemed to kill the fungus and the hole would heal up from the bottom, although it took a long time and the sores were very painful. Teeth also were affected; gums receded and teeth fell out – a form of gingivitis. Rosie's teeth became so bad that she had to be sent home for treatment and did not return to us until we reached France. Ascorbic acid, which had to be taken daily, helped. We also had to take a daily dose of atebrin against malaria and, when the temperature rose above 100°F, a tablespoon of salt.

The NAAFI at Tobruk supplied us with our monthly ration of extras. There we could buy whisky for eight shillings a bottle, and gin for six shillings. We could also buy beer, toothpaste, boot polish, soap, razor blades and unique cigarettes called 'Victory', made in India from goodness knows what, and came in packets of 20 in a purple carton with a large 'V' stamped on each side. Occasionally we were lucky and drew Players or Craven A, which came in useful round tins of 50. Few of the Quakers drank or smoked but we drew their rations just the same – which made us very popular with the Division as we always had a good supply of alcohol and cigarettes to offer them. The French took to whisky and porridge as if they were Scottish born and we took to wine with the same enthusiasm. No Frenchman can exist without his 'pinard' any more than an Englishman can without his tea, so wherever we were we always had wine and tea.

There was an extraordinary comradeship and true brotherhood during the whole of the Western desert campaign. To belong to and be part of the Eighth Army was a passport to anywhere, irrespective of colour, race, creed or sex. The campaign ribbon, the 'Desert Star' (more commonly called the 'Desert Sore') was the most sought-after decoration and to qualify one had to have been in the desert before the Battle of El Alamein. If one was lucky enough to be part of that brotherhood everything that was theirs was yours. If your vehicle broke down someone would come along and help, or if you were short of a spare part or a drink from a water bottle, or needed a lift by road or air, you only had to ask. It was your right as part of the Eighth Army.

Of course there was, as well, a certain amount of unofficial scrounging between units. If someone could 'make' an extra piece of equipment, good luck to them. Most of the regiments in the desert possessed far more than their official number of vehicles and panic ensued when an inspection was announced. The extra 'bits' were hastily hidden away or garaged with another unit until the inspection was over. Occasionally the scrounging went too far as, for example, when a top general's staff car was acquired by a squadron and had to be surreptitiously returned before the theft was discovered.

When the Eighth Army was split up at the end of the desert campaign this camaraderie was never regained. We went back to divisions and units, each for himself. We were told the reason it was reorganised before it reached Italy was because it had such insufferable pride and conceit when it met up with the First Army in Tunisia.

The war had advanced to Tripolitania and Stukas no long dive-bombed us. The Division was *en repos* re-equipping and training new recruits. Our wadi, now that it had stopped raining, no longer drowned us. It led down to the sea – clean golden sand and calm blue sea. We bathed whenever we had a moment and held parties there. Evelyn's gramophone was much in demand. Our old friend, the First Armoured

Division – known as the Rhinos because of their badge – which consisted of (among others) the Queen's Bays, Kit's brother John's regiment and other cavalry regiments always seemed to be stationed near us. I knew several of them before the war.

The French also paid us visits, the Foreign Legion, the Fusilier Marin, Artillery and all the regiments of foot. The Colonel and Lady Spears both gave parties. May was particularly fond of the 11th Hussars, her husband's old regiment, in which we had several friends. Of course we were spoilt; there were no other women in the desert at that time and very few in Egypt, so we were much in demand and it was difficult not to get one's head turned.

A few days later we received orders that the Division was moving *en bloc* to a destination unknown but somewhere beyond Tripoli, with the hope of going into battle again at the Mareth line.

We started out at midday on 18 April 1943 on what was to be our longest convoy of the war – over 1,000 vehicles – and reached Maturba, our camp, that first night at 8pm. The First Brigade was a day ahead of us, followed by the Second Brigade, then us followed by the Atelier Lourd to pick up stragglers and breakdowns. We were very short of drivers in the Hospital and all the officers who could drive were given a vehicle. We drivers took over the water buggies again, in addition to our staff cars. I drove 82, which by this time had become 'my car', and had the sisters Edith Irving and Betty Corthay as my passengers. The clobber the Nannies expected us to carry for them was unbelievable and there were always rows when we refused to accept some of their larger items – insisting that they either went in the luggage truck or were thrown away. They seemed to be particularly attached to empty shell cases and ammunition boxes and had baskets crammed with surplus possessions which they could not get into their trunks. On convoy our usually smart staff cars looked more like gypsy caravans, with bundles of flea bags tied to their roof racks and water bottles and more bundles hanging down from them. The Nannies were not the only guilty ones – Barbara, on this convoy, had a tea chest tied to the back of her car containing her two pigeons which, at the last moment, inconsiderately laid two eggs and started to sit on them – quite a feat during the bumping in the heat and the dust. She let them out each evening when we arrived at our destination to fly around. They always returned and, to everyone's surprise, hatched out their chicks on the day we reached 'Marble Arch'.

The convoy was rigorously disciplined. Divisional police on fast motor cycles rushed up and down the line of vehicles like sheep dogs, reporting on bad driving and distances incorrectly kept. The rule was 20 yards between each vehicle, no more no less. General Brosset, too, generally paid us a daily visit to see how we were progressing. Our section of the convoy of some 60 vehicles was led as usual by Mike

Rowntree in his 'Biscuit Tin'. We also had our own scouts on motor cycles to help and encourage us. We also had to keep well into the right side of the road, which was difficult with all the pot-holes and craters.

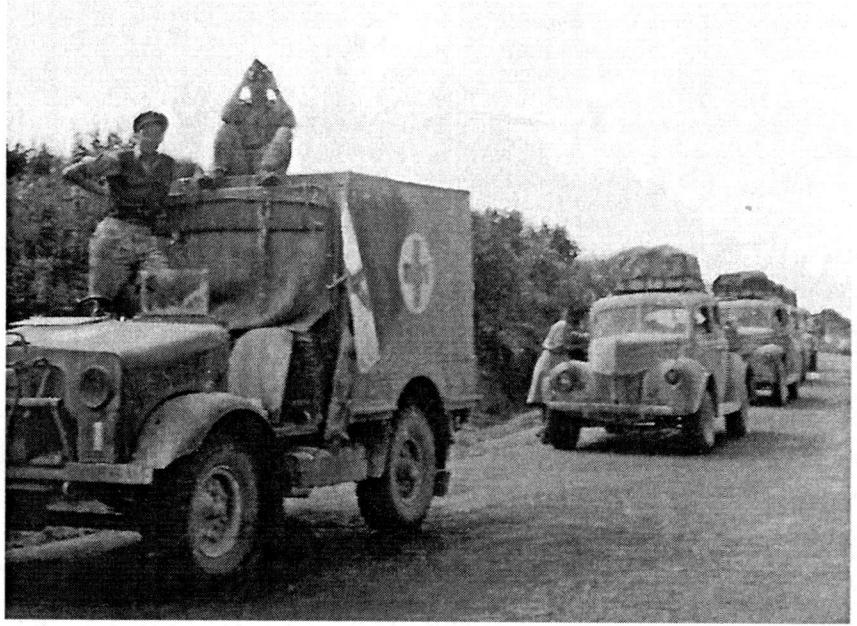

Michael Rowntree leads the convoy in his Biscuit Tin.

We were scheduled to have a ten-minute halt every two hours and a half hour break for lunch and supper. Our ten-minute halts seldom worked out but we did appreciate them when they occurred. We all suffered in varying degrees from driver's cramp and the breaks gave us a chance to stretch our legs and wake up.

We drove at 20mph when we were on our own, but the official speed of the divisional convoy was 16mph. This was cruel to our staff cars, which were built for speed. They were seldom out of third gear and, with the sand and dust thrown up by the trucks in front, continually boiled over in spite of their condensers. The overheated oil caused them to seize up and we fell by the wayside, thus losing our place in the convoy. When we got going again, we were not supposed to pass anything except halted vehicles. We did, of course, and hoped we would be mistaken for an important general; it was a pleasant change to drive at speed again.

The straight desert roads with nothing but sand to look at were so monotonous that you became hypnotised by the car in front and after long hours of driving it became increasingly difficult to concentrate on keeping the correct distance and not fall asleep. Vehicles frequently and suddenly careered drunkenly across the road. When this happened everyone blew their horns hoping to awaken the driver before he bumped into someone or ran off the road. Sudden halts often caused collisions. One day we came to rather an abrupt halt and I was just about to take a swig from my water bottle when we sprang a few yards further up the road with a bang which reminded us that there were still a few mines left in the road – but no, the car behind us had not noticed that we had stopped.

We were all very well organised with rations for the convoy drive and there was always a hot meal ready waiting for us by the time we bivouacked for the night however late we arrived. The cooks had an odd-looking kitchen on wheels in a trailer which didn't break down during the whole war. They were adept at producing thick hot stews at night and a curious beverage which called itself 'coffee' in the mornings and 'tea' at night. It was hot, strong and very sweet and we were grateful for it.

We pulled off the road for our first night beyond Maturba and bivouacked in an uneven circle. We gulped down our hot stew and tea, pulled our sleeping bags out and settled down for the night. Some of us had wirelesses and we listened to the news and *Lily Marlene* (the German army song) before going to sleep.

The singing of the birds and crickets woke us up at daybreak and after a breakfast of hot porridge, army biscuits, jam, margarine and coffee we packed up our bedding, got ourselves in line and waited for the order to move off. We were always ready long before we received our instructions for the day, but it was pleasant lying in the early morning sun, reading or listening to the wireless.

Our second day's driving took us through the fertile land of Cyrenaica, and after our eight months in Egypt and the desert it was like the promised land of the Israelites to us. In Roman times it was called the Granary of Europe.

Derna, the gateway to this paradise, is approached by a very steep twisting hill and lies in a deep hollow. It was a beautiful and unexpected sight, appearing suddenly as we rounded a bend in the road. The sea encircling the bay was a deep aquamarine with the sky of the same colour reaching down to meet it. Dazzling white buildings surrounded the bay, tall houses with gardens bright with flowers, bougainvillea climbed the walls, and peach and almond trees in blossom lined the streets. Derna appeared to have escaped the worst of the war and for the first time in our drive we saw both Italians and Arabs walking the streets.

The road leading from Derna followed the coast for a while and then climbed steeply away from the sea. The landscape from here was richly green, the sand of the desert disappeared completely and was replaced by a deep red soil. We passed farm houses and saw Italian farmers busy working their land with the help of mules and horses.

They had a few cows and some scraggy sheep and goats. As we continued further into Cyrenaica enclosed fields of corn become more numerous with orchards of olive and fruit trees surrounded by tall poplar trees.

Every twenty kilometres or so we drove past a collection of buildings, always the same shape and size, one-storey houses painted white with green windows and doors, farm buildings, and a church, school, mairie and market with '*Ente Colonizzio Lybia*' inscribed on an archway. We were warned not to enter any Italian buildings as most of the empty ones had been mined or booby-trapped by the retreating Italians.

Once we had left the perimeter of Derna we saw less and less livestock. We were told that the Germans had requisitioned and slaughtered all they could lay their hands on and that the Bedouin had stolen and hidden away any that remained, while their owners were hiding from the battles.

Though we rarely saw any signs of poultry all the way to Tunisia, each time we halted, Arab children arrived from nowhere shouting 'Eggies' and displaying pigeon-sized eggs in baskets or tied in old bits of cloth. They offered them in exchange for cigarettes, tea or anything else they could get. The usual barter was one egg for three cigarettes or a handful of tea. The least complicated way of dealing with an egg was to tie it in a handkerchief and drop it into the radiator of a car, which was usually at boiling point. In a few minutes one had an *œuf a la coq* which, providing it was not bad, was a pleasant change from army rations.

On this second day's journey we did not arrive at our destination until well after dark. It was bitterly cold and we wrapped ourselves in every available covering, sleeping as usual beside our cars. We were not too pleased to be woken up next morning by General Brosset who was dressed immaculately in pressed shorts and bush shirt and apparently not feeling the cold at all. He announced that he was staying to breakfast.

Cyrenaica, hilly, green and fertile, continued until Benghazi when we came upon deep gorges covered in trees and streams of clear water rushing and skipping over rocks and moss-covered stones. What a delight! That day we drove through D'Annuncio, Madelina Baracca, Barce Oriano and Barce, the most delightful towns with mimosa and fruit trees in blossom everywhere. Everywhere was green, and bordering the road from town to town were wild gladioli, lupins, poppies and flowers of every colour.

Soon after leaving Barce the road descended through a long winding escarpment which took us to sea level again. Almost immediately the vegetation became sparser and thinner and the red earth changed to pale sand. The Italian farms and buildings became fewer and fewer and for the first time we passed large encampments of Bedouin with herds of goats, sheep, camels and horses.

Benghazi was a gloomy town surrounded by dirty grey sand littered with rubbish and all the agglomeration of war. We by-passed most of it and continued for another 20 kilometres before halting near an Arab enclosure. Here we remained for a day's rest and maintenance of the vehicles.

The next morning we spent servicing our cars. It was very hot and the dirty, grey, powdery sand got into our eyes, ears and hair. Adding to our discomfort fleas and flies attacked us with venom. By lunch time we had finished our work and we all rushed off to the beach at Sîwa to try and clean the worst of the dirt from our bodies and hair and to escape the insect attacks. In the evening we wandered round the bazaars of Benghazi where junk of every description was offered for sale, including gaudy postcards and handkerchiefs printed with the bull-necked face of Mussolini grinning into the impassive face of Hitler.

Our next day of convoy driving started at the late hour of 11am and took us to about 40 miles beyond Agebadia. Our whole trek was 1,538 miles, and we averaged between 150 and 200 miles a day.

Agebadia was the scene of a fierce and bitter tank battle during the Eighth Army advance against Rommel. The battlefield had been cleared up by the time we passed through; the wrecked tanks, guns, aeroplanes and trucks had been piled into huge dumps. This day's drive was particularly unpleasant; the temperature increased noticeably and the air felt heavy and oppressive. Quite suddenly a hot wind blew in from the Sahara, whipping up the sand and bringing with it a fine dust which penetrated everywhere. The cars kept boiling over, their condensers seemed to make no difference.

We dipped our water bottles in water and hung them out of the windows to try and keep them cool but the water evaporated too quickly even though they had felt covers. The dust even got through their screw tops. The roads were wet with liquid tar which squelched under the tyres as we drove along. The sand and dust got into our eyes and made them smart, but wearing the goggles we had been given was even worse. They stuck to sweat on our faces and burnt our skins and the dust got in under them in spite of the rubber surface. The sand blotted out the sun but it made no difference to the heat. Only when the sun went down did the wind abate. We were thankful when we reached our leaguer for the night.

The following day's drive was hot but without the wind and sand. We drove through Mersa, Birga and Al Agaila, stopping for the night at

Ras El Aali just beyond the frontier into Tripolitania. One of our halts was beside 'Marble Arch', the triumphal arch erected by Mussolini to glorify his colonial possessions and conquest in Northern Africa. Built of marble and towering over the barren desert, it is a splendid piece of architecture. High up over the arch is a bronze figure of a Roman runner whose legend was learnt by every schoolchild in Mussolini's day. Inscribed in Latin above the bronze figure are the words: 'O Sun, you will never see a town like Rome'.

The legend of the Roman runner is as follows: in ancient times the Romans and Carpathians, wishing to settle once and for all the dispute over the frontier, agreed to each send a runner from the farthest end of their respective countries and wherever they met the boundary would be fixed. The Roman ran with such speed that he covered twice the distance of the Carpathian runner and met him well inside the Carpathian country. The Carpathians accused the Romans of cheating, whereupon the Roman athlete drew his sword and killed himself to prove his innocence, thereby winning the boundary in Rome's favour.

The eighth day was the longest drive of the journey and started very early in the morning. 206 miles brought us to Sultan where we rested for 24 hours on scrubby waste land overlooking the sea. We went to sleep with the sound of the sea in our ears and the promise of a bathe next day.

The next day was Easter Sunday. We did not even know this until Mass was followed by a double ration of pinard, produced for us by the indefatigable Père Boileau. Sultan is in the Gulf of Sirte. We learnt how treacherous the sea is there; our strongest swimmers ventured out from the rest of us and were held there by a powerful undercurrent. Eventually a human chain of about 50 swimmers holding hands succeeded in reaching them after – what seemed to us watching from the shore – an agonisingly long time. They were all safely rescued.

We continued on our way on Easter Monday, driving through mile after mile of sand, rock and dust with nothing to break the monotony except a flying column of Greek Commandos, 'The Immortals', who looked even scruffier than we did. They scorched past us with tattered beards and bloodshot eyes, their sweat and sand-ingrained faces the colour of American Indians. We drove straight through Sirte which was badly damaged with most of the palm trees that had lined the streets lying broken or with their trunks split in two. We halted for the night near Buerat beside a large salt lake where duck and flamingo were flighting into the twilight. The mosquitoes rose in hordes as the sun went down and even our mosquito nets, which were difficult to hang from our cars, were small protection from them. The sunrise next morning was glorious and we lay, half asleep, watching the birds rising and descending in flocks, pink-winged flamingos, many different species of wild duck, including the whistling widgeon, and skeins of sand geese in perfect formation and honking as they flew past us.

We struck the road again at 9.30 on Tuesday, driving through many Italian towns. The Italians had returned to their houses now that the war was over for them. They were ragged and pathetic; the women all wore large straw hats and the children were barefoot and in tattered clothes. The only difference between them and the Arab children was that they did not beg or shout 'Baksheesh' at us, though many of the adults asked us for cigarettes.

Misratah, near where we stopped for the night, lived up to its name. Half Arab, half Italian, timidly cultivated with sparse wheat and barley clinging to the shade of the palm trees, a few plantains were scattered through the silvery sand and bright green irises. Kit made friends with an Arab boy and he brought her a little grey yearling colt to ride. It had a cruel bit in its mouth and a huge saddle covered in velvet and richly embroidered. The stirrups were rather a let-down – they had been cut out of a petrol can.

We were glad when we left this part of the desert; it was so bare and desolate and each side of the road was heavily mined.

We left Misratah on 28 April, the eleventh day of the convoy. It should have been our last, but when we reached our leaguer for the night we were told that we were to push on over the Tunisian frontier to the front line. Our Division was to relieve the New Zealanders who had had very heavy casualties. The French were pleased and a new sense of urgency inspired the convoy drivers. No one was going to be left behind and whatever went wrong with their vehicles they somehow managed to limp on, even if it was at the end of a rope.

Beyond Misratah the desert receded: less sand and scrub, more cultivation, cleaner, neater houses, more prosperity. We stopped for lunch near the Roman ruins of Leptis Magna but had no time to visit them. After driving through Homs it became very hot indeed and the cars all began to boil over and seize up. Iris fell by the wayside with a leaking radiator and had to be towed. At Homs we turned away from the sea and drove over very badly rutted roads and tracks into more hilly country with a range of hills in the distance, green with trees. We halted for the night in an olive grove beyond Breviglera.

Because of the need to reach the battle zone as soon as possible our daily average had been pushed up to 300 kilometres, but we still had to travel at the speed of the slowest vehicle. This made a long day's drive.

We continued through several small Italian towns and back to the coast again, through Sabratha (more Roman ruins), Zuara and Pirida and over the Tunisian frontier at Ben Gardane and to about 60 miles beyond. Parts of the road were very bad indeed and slowed the heavy trucks down to 10mph. This had a disastrous effect on our staff cars. They started to boil over again and stall. The dust kicked up from the tracks by the heavies played havoc with our carburettors and petrol pumps, which we frequently had to take to bits and clean. It was dark by the time we drove through Ben Gardane and I was having trouble with 82. Apart from over-heating and stalling the self-starter kept on jamming and eventually packed up altogether. Her lights and horn had failed as well. I managed to keep on the road by driving on the tail of the car in front of me, which gave me just enough light to see the edge of the road. A push from behind got me going again each time the car stalled. We reached our leaguer very late at night and very tired. We were on the road again next morning after getting up at five to service and clean out the entire petrol system of our cars. Half our hospital was missing when we halted and lorries came limping in all night – many, like Iris, on the end of a tow rope. Nevertheless, everything which could move was in line next morning for the final lap. A better road and cooler temperature helped a lot.

We drove through Medenine, a very curious town with beehive houses, one on top of another on the side of a cliff. Now that we were on French soil again we got a few cheers as we drove through the narrow streets of small towns. Through Mareth, which had been almost completely destroyed, Gabès, a large garrison town, and Metabes where we forked to the right and continued along a very small, narrow road and spent the night on sandy soil in an olive grove. We celebrated our arrival in a French colony by drinking sweet champagne, produced by Père Boileau who had lovingly hoarded it for just this occasion.

There were no orders for us the following morning so we took advantage of the rest to repair the most urgent disorders of our vehicles. Our orders arrived next day – we were no longer part of the Division convoy. We were to proceed to 20 kilometres north of Sousse to Sidi Bou Ali, where the New Zealand CCS had prepared a site for us alongside their hospital and as near as possible to the front line where we would receive the wounded from our Division when they attacked.

We started off in columns of eight. This was necessary because of the build-up of military traffic on the narrow roads. We by-passed Triago and drove through Hamman, Djennual and Sousse to Sidi Bou Ali. Our final destination was on top of a small hill under a few olive trees within five miles of the sea, which we could clearly see in the distance. We were thankful to have arrived at last. The Division had completed 2,400 miles in 15 days with three days of *repos*.

5

VICTORY IN NORTH AFRICA

The hospital tents were immediately erected among the olive trees, well scattered in case of air attacks. It consequently took us some time and much walking to find our way around. From the time we arrived, continuous waves of aeroplanes (mostly allied fighters and bombers) flew over, sometimes more than 100, on their way to help with the final attack on the German lines. They flew chiefly at sunrise and sunset and looked like silver fish as the sun glinted on their wings. There was a good deal of gunfire and the 'crump, crump' of exploding shells, together with bright flashes, which became louder and clearer at night, could be heard and seen not many miles away.

The following morning, 7 May 1942, we all helped to put the hospital into working order, cutting up swabs, dressings and plaster bandages in readiness for the arrival of the wounded. After lunch we were given a few hours off duty and Kit, Biddy and I accepted an invitation from the New Zealanders to ride their mules. We thought it would be easy – like riding donkeys on the Margate sands. We hadn't bargained for mule saddles, lumps of stuffing in a sack with a body belt to secure them and no stirrups. Every time a mule put his head down, which he did frequently, saddle and rider tipped forward and down the neck in slow motion – to the amusement of the onlookers.

The same day the division moved up to a forward position near Enfidaville relieving the New Zealanders. The Germans and Italians were firmly entrenched on an escarpment at Zaghouan, which was a natural defence.

A forward hospital unit under Captain Thibaux aided by Lieutenants Albert and Schick, with five members of the Friends' Ambulance Unit and several Senegalese orderlies was sent to the front-line near Takrouna behind the attacking line. We gave them a farewell party on the eve of their departure. They remained there from until 14 May and, although they were shelled several times, neither they nor their wounded were hit. We could see the battle taking place quite clearly from our hill top but were soon too busy to find time to watch.

Our main hospital received casualties between 9 May and 5 June. During particularly heavy fighting between 12 and 20 May we received 130 casualties each day; the rest of the time it was between 70 and 80 a day. To accommodate newcomers we had to evacuate the same number to British base hospitals.

The staff of the New Zealand hospital below our hill were very hospitable. Among other things, they offered us the use of their hot showers; we accepted with alacrity for (except on leave) we had not had this luxury since leaving Egypt. It was amazing how our skins changed colour with the help of soap and hot water. What we had imagined was sun tan turned out to be a mixture of motor oil and dirt. Our hair also benefited from a change of shampoo – soap instead of paraffin. They invited us to watch the film *Desert Victory* with them – a curious experience, seated on the ground in the open air at night with our own planes flying overhead and with the noise and barrage of the battle a few miles away – some 500 people packed into tidy rows with bright cinema lights on the screen and not an enemy plane to bother us. We relived the Western Desert campaign and enjoyed seeing the familiar faces and places again.

Bizerte and Tunis were liberated on 7 May 1942 but the fighting continued more intensely than ever over the next few days. On 9 May wounded arrived all through the night; everybody was up helping. In the morning I was told to open a new ward for the overflow. The tent was put up and, as there were no beds left, I collected as many stretchers and blankets as I could lay my hands on and tried to beg, borrow or steal the necessary equipment. My help consisted of one FAU orderly, and two African orderlies. I ended the day with 30 wounded, among them several German and Italian prisoners who all admitted that the war in North Africa was virtually over. I hoped that they were right.

The forward hospital unit returned on 14 May, providing more help in the main hospital. They had many stories to tell, including one about our own tirailleurs who wanted to murder all the wounded prisoners. They also told us the horrifying tale of more than 100 Frenchmen captured wearing German uniform, most of them from Alsace and Lorraine. But for the presence of British troops they would certainly have been shot by the French soldiers – and some were.

By the end of the month the tempo of the hospital had slowed and most of the patients in my ward had been evacuated. I had only a few slightly wounded left and so was able to snatch a few hours off duty. One morning an Arab arrived at my tent riding one horse and leading another and offered them to me to ride in exchange for tins of bully beef and cigarettes. Riding a horse around the countryside was the best way of sightseeing and Kit and I were delighted. We went for many rides through a green valley dotted with white houses, and olive trees planted with meticulous care in straight rows. We rode through fields of maize, barley and wheat divided by hedges of cactus. The Arab also gave us mare's milk to drink which was very good and slightly sweet.

The insect life continued to plague us. One day Biddy and I found a deserted hut and brought out of it two useful earthenware pitchers for water. As we left I said to Biddy: 'We had better look out for creepy crawlies'; then, looking down at my legs I saw, to my horror, that they were black with fleas. We dropped the pitchers and flew back to our tent where we tore off our clothes, covered ourselves with DDT and soaked our clothes in petrol. However, not all insects attacked us. Scarab and dung beetles were amusing to watch, rolling their balls of mud and dung around. So were the scorpions as long as we kept well away from them. We used to keep praying mantis in our tents and occasionally we found a chameleon and made him change colour by putting him on different coloured backgrounds. There were also snakes, lizards and tortoises.

Now that the war in North Africa was over it was amusing to note the increase in livestock. Horses, sheep and goats appeared from nowhere – and even cattle, which had been cleverly hidden by the French and Arab farmers, became a common sight. There were not many birds around; perhaps the noise of battle had frightened them away. There were a few larks and a strange bird resembling an outsize wagtail, which flitted from tree to tree making a noise like an animal in pain. We saw an occasional golden oriole (a beautiful bird) and several hoopoes, comical when they displayed their crests.

Lady Spears turned up in the middle of May, a few days after the Tunisian war had ended. She approved of our site at Sidi Bou Ali, which was very pleasant. We had put our tents near olive trees for shade. Tunisia in May was not unbearably hot, the days were sunny and the nights cool. At the time of her visit wounded had stopped arriving and the wards were only half full. Lady Spears was delighted with the work the forward unit had done and with the hospital itself. Madame Catroux, the wife of General Catroux, turned up while when she was with us and did a tour of the hospital with the Colonel. She was rude to some of the wounded who had joined us from the Vichy regiments in North Africa; Lady Spears was not amused.

Lady Spears stayed with us only a few days and when she left we were all given leave to go to Tunis or elsewhere within driving distance. I chose Tunis, which proved to be a great disappointment. There were very few shops open and everything was very expensive. The RAF had completely flattened the docks with their accurate bombing, although the town had escaped with only a little damage.

One of the difficulties which caused trouble between the First Army and the Eighth in Tunisia was the question of dress. The First Army

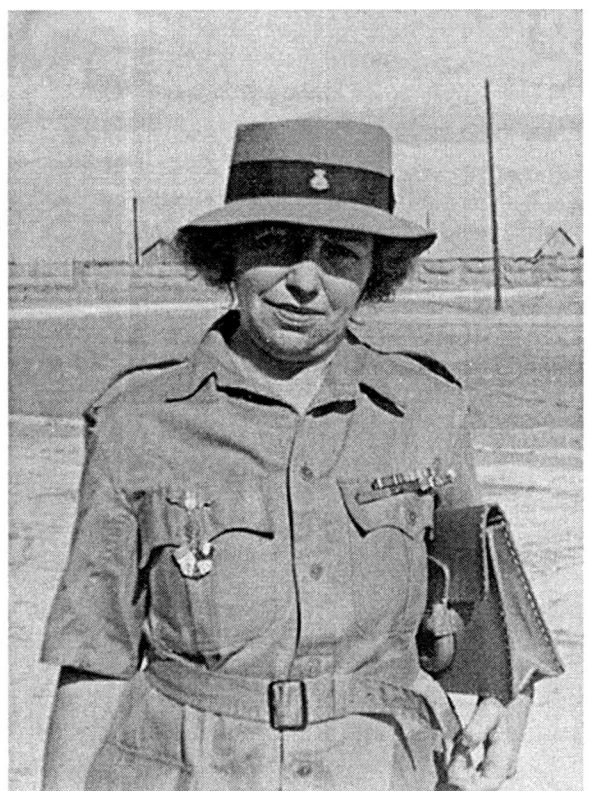

Lady Spears.

arrived in immaculate starched and pressed shorts, starched shirts, neat stockings, highly polished black boots and gleaming leather belts. The Eighth Army wore their own things – baggy corduroy trousers (which had usually seen better days) or shorts down to their knees, bush shirts, desert boots and coloured silk scarves around their necks. When it became chilly they wore a curious collection of khaki jerseys (reaching below their knees) or Arab sheepskin coats which stank to high heaven. They usually carried an Arab fly whisk to ward off the hordes of flies, and very often a tin mug or can was attached to their belt. The two 'types' were brilliantly depicted by 'Jon' in the *Eighth Army News* cartoons.

Another bone of contention was rations. The First Army was issued with tins of either Craven A or Players cigarettes whereas we had to make do with the disgusting V cigarettes. Their beer was bottled while ours was tinned and they had jeeps which were new to us and much coveted.

A few days after the fall of Tunis we met up with the First Army who had worked their way down to us from Algeria and Morocco. They appeared to be a very different species from the Eighth Army. Apart from the difference in dress code there was also quite a bit of jealousy and ill-feeling in other areas. Each claimed to have reached Tunis first. The First Army thought we were insufferably arrogant (which we were) and we envied them their newer equipment and better rations. We also felt that the First Army MPs went out of their way to harass us and I fear we were pretty off-hand with them all.

It was at this time that a First Army officer brought an American jeep to our hospital and gave us a demonstration. He drove it straight through a cactus hedge with no ill effects and over bumps and humps that no ordinary lorry or car could negotiate. It was the first 4-wheel drive we had seen. We were very impressed and envious and determined to get one for ourselves.

With so much friction between the two armies there were inevitably fights which resulted in some blood and even a death or two. There was also trouble of a much more serious kind between us. The Free French and the French troops stationed in North Africa who had been there since the French armistice with the Germans in 1941. Many of them had fought against the American and British troops when they landed in North Africa in November 1942. The Moustachios, or Giraudists as the Free French called them, were under the command of Admiral Darlan and, after Darlan's assassination, General Giraud.

The political temperature concerning the French forces and the struggle between de Gaulle and Giraud for supremacy was reflected in the mutual suspicion between the two. Another reason for friction was the number of soldiers deserting from the North African regiments to join our Division which, after all, had been fighting the Germans since the fall of France.

We knew nothing of the high politics being played in Algiers between Giraud (backed by the Americans) and de Gaulle (backed by the British), but the entire Division was furious when we received the order to leave Tunisia and go back down the desert to Zuara in Tripolitania, one of the hottest places in Africa. Banished with us was the Colonne Leclerc. I watched part of it arrive. I saw a vehicle pulling two others. Looking more like a gypsy caravan than an army, it had travelled up from Fort Lamy in Chad on its own wheels, traversing the Sahara Desert to join the Eighth Army and take part in the final attack on Tunisia.

The Free French never understood this strange decision expelling them from a French colony they had fought so gallantly since 1941 to reach. To say that they were embittered was an understatement; they felt rejected and disgraced and the bitterness between the two armies continued until the campaign in Italy was over.

5 June – We receive orders to pack up the hospital and be ready to move on. The hospital is only half full and by evening all the patients

have been evacuated to hospitals in Sousse and Tunis, and the tents start coming down. The cars are serviced and cleaned out.

7 June – Our own tents are taken down and we spend the night in the open. At daybreak little bands of Arabs turn up to see what pickings are left for them. We keep a sharp guard on the cars (and our belongings) as we load up.

8 June – I drive Barbara and one Nanny – Betty Corthay. We, and the Colonel, with Aboucher, set off ahead of the convoy to the ordnance depot and civilian hospital at Sfax. We eat our lunch near the sea outside Sfax and pick up the convoy on a very dusty road between Triaga and Keriouan. We continue with them for about thirty miles and then halt for the night at the identical spot we bivouacked in on our way up.

9 June – A long and dusty drive on our own, not with the rest of the Division. We make good time and the roads on the whole are good. We do 160 miles in the day. After miles of sandy desert we halted for lunch at the Oasis of Gabès, which must surely be one of the most beautiful and one of the most written about from the time of Pliny the younger to today. Tall palm and mimosa trees give shade and protection to apricot and fig trees around, under which grow vines, flowers and vegetables in rich profusion. Sparkling clear water winds its way through this Garden of Eden ending in a large pool where children play and women wash their clothes, and flocks of camel, sheep and goats drink their fill. Alas, we leave it far too quickly to return to the desert sand and heat, though our road does take us near enough to the sea to catch a sea breeze. Through Medinine, the curious Arab town with houses built like beehives into the side of the cliffs. Girls covered in jewellery watch as the convoy winds its way through the narrow streets, children play and men wearing burnouses and smoking hubble-bubble pipes sit outside on the pavements. We drive on to Ben Gardane – a French garrison town – and through the Mareth line and stop for the night under a few scrubby fig trees.

10 June – Off again after an excellent breakfast of eggs (bought from the Arabs the night before), bacon and coffee prepared by Barbara. We halt for the night on the far side of Zelten, driving off the road and up a track between two Italian houses and five minutes' walk to the sea. We arrive in daylight and Barbara and I walk back to the houses and talk to the Italians living there. They seemed pleased to see us and gave us hot water and eggs for breakfast.

11 June – We stayed at this camp for 24 hours while the Colonel and Barbara went off to find a permanent site. Time to service and repair our cars and clean ourselves with a bathe in the sea.

12 June – We drive to our new site, only a few miles away in a marvellous position, well away from the road across a salt flat. This is hard and dry and within a few yards of the sea with cliffs leading down to the seashore. Plenty of room for the hospital tents and our own, which we pitch to the left of the hospital and as close to the sea as we can put them. There is some doubt as to whether we will be allowed to stay here for long. General Relanger, the Chief Medical Officer at the French Headquarters, does not approve of our choice. However, everyone is busy helping to put up the tents and our first patients arrived that afternoon.

We stayed at this site until the beginning of September. We soon discovered that we were only a few miles from a pleasant little town called Zuara and quite near the Roman ruins of Sabratha. During this period the hospital was not very busy. We were given a generous amount of time off and we all had a week's leave and permission to spend it anywhere we could arrange in the Middle East.

Both the British First Armoured Division and the Eighth Armoured Brigade were stationed near Tripoli and we saw a lot of them, as well as a squadron of RAF fighter friends of Jocelyn's. In fact there seemed to be an endless round of parties and weekends in Tripoli. The Free French in London managed to send out Germaine Sablon, who had escaped from France over the Pyrenees with other French artistes, to entertain us. They gave a concert in the Roman theatre at Sabratha and Germaine sang the famous *Chant des Partisans*, the song of the French Resistance. She decided to remain with us and was a great help to the wounded and distributed Red Cross comforts to them.

Tripoli at this time housed the Area Headquarters, the Paymaster General, an Officers' shop, the NAAFI and a bank, so we were always being sent there on errands. It was a pleasant town. The largest hotel, the Del Mahari, was an officers' hotel and club. It served cheap army food and drink and had clean bedrooms with hot and cold running water. The baths were square with curious square seats which made it impossible to lie down in them and difficult to fill with enough water for comfort. However, they were a welcome change from the tin basin and jerry can of the desert. In Tripoli there was also a very efficiently run YWCA which served better food and had pleasanter rooms, but no alcohol. We generally stayed there and were allowed to invite officers to meals. We always had a queue of them hoping for an invitation. We also spent many happy hours wandering through the Arab quarters in the market square, bargaining at length for anything that caught our fancy. A month after we arrived General de Gaulle paid the hospital his only visit. He made himself unpopular by keeping us waiting for three hours, lined up on the salt flats, under a scorching sun.

At the beginning of July we experienced a terrible heatwave and sandstorm. It had been gradually building up during the previous week and lasted for three miserable days. The temperature soared to 125°F in the shade and there was little of that in the desert. Inside the tents it was stifling. The mercury in the clinical thermometers rushed to the top and broke them. A hot fog-like wind, laden with fine particles of sand, blew mercilessly day and night. Sand got into everything – food, water, hair, ears and eyes. With no escape we felt we would go mad. It was impossible to sleep at night and when we were not on duty we spent the time in the tepid sea. We realised how lucky we were to be so near the sea compared to the rest of the Division. We attached our water bottles and cans of beer to rocks in the sea in an attempt to cool them and then forgot where we had put them. The hospital patients suffered most of all, lying in their sweat-drenched sheets, stiff with sand. Several of them were in plaster under which the sand crept and irritated. Driving our cars was torture. We burnt our hands on the steering wheels and had to wear gloves. Metal was too hot to touch, cans of petrol exploded and the car radiators boiled over every few miles in spite of the condensers and driving them as fast as they would go. The fierce wind cracked our lips and burnt our skins. The rubber goggles we were given (to protect our eyes when we drove) stuck to our skin and scalded it. Even walking in the sand was painful; the heat burnt through the soles of our desert boots.

We were lucky that the khamseen lasted only three days. It can often last as long as seven days by which time most people have gone mad. As it was, during the heatwave Joan Pryke and Jocelyn Russell were attacked while asleep by an unknown French soldier. Joan was sleeping outside her tent in her flea-bag; he attacked her first, trying to roll her out of it, but she shouted and fought him off. He then tried Jocelyn, who was the only one of us sleeping alone in a very small bell tent (which had been given to me by the RAF and which we took turns to use) and attempted to get under her mosquito net. In doing so he woke her up. She explained politely to him, in her very individual French, that she was a married woman. He was so astonished by this surprising argument that he gave up the attempt and disappeared. We never found out which regiment he came from; the upshot was that more guards were put on night duty and we were made to sleep two or more in a tent and forbidden to sleep in the open.

During this banishment to Tripolitania our Free French division was badly fed and equipped. While the Generals and Politicians argued about whether we were to be under the command of the British or the

Americans we became 'nobody's children'. Our petrol was cut down and our rations reduced. Even our Syrian cooks ran out of ideas of what to do with bully beef. This lack of variety in our diet had a very bad effect on everyone's health – we all suffered from vitamin deficiency even though we took daily pills of ascorbic acid. Desert sores increased and became really troublesome and we all suffered to some degree from conjunctivitis, bleeding teeth and receding gums.

To cheer us up someone had the bright idea of sending two of our four water buggies to Tunisia to fill them with cheap red wine; unobtainable in Tripolitania and without which no self-respecting Frenchman will work or fight. Unfortunately, they forgot that the tanks were lined with zinc, and by the time they returned triumphantly the wine had eaten through it. The wine was undrinkable and the tanks were ruined; we had to send all the way to Cairo for replacements.

During our *repos* in Tripolitania we were given ten days' leave. My turn began on 4 August and I decided to spend it in Egypt. At 5am Biddy drove me to the RAF airport outside Tripoli at Castel Benito. I hopped a lift on an old Douglas transport plane. There were 30 of us on board, packed like sardines and perched on small tin plates facing each other.

Although we flew at only 10,000 feet it was bitterly cold after the heat of the desert. There was no heating and everyone was dressed in thin drill uniform. I was lucky in being the only woman; the pilot invited me into the warm cockpit. On the way he pointed out the recent battle areas. One could see plainly all the vehicle tracks and the mine fields, still marked, and it was easy to comprehend the way the battles had ebbed and flowed. After a stop at Benghazi we touched down at Mena airport, a few miles outside Cairo, where our luggage was searched for silks, furs and narcotics – or so they said. I wondered where we could have got such things. After this indignity we were driven in a bus and deposited outside Shepheard's Hotel. To my dismay I discovered that a room which should have been booked for me was not available; luckily Vera and Ted Sanders kindly put me up. The first thing I did was to have a long, deep bath, after which my ten days' leave passed quickly in a wonderful round of riding, racing, tennis, squash and swimming at the Ghezera Club with dinners at the Mohammed Club and the Turf Club. So many friends of mine were on leave at the same time that every night I went dancing at the numerous night clubs, two of which were outside Cairo on the road to the pyramids, the *Auberge des Pyramides* and the *Chasse Royale* where they shot pigeons during the daytime. Both were owned by King Farouk who was generally to be seen each night at one or the other – fat, florid and surrounded by dancing girls.

During this leave I got into trouble with Army Intelligence and was lucky not to have been put into 'protective custody' as it was then called. I was back living in Shepheard's Hotel where one evening I was having dinner with George Jellicoe, Vivian Street and several others – all in the SAS. They had just returned from Syria where they had been training and practising parachute jumps, and were being mysterious and irritating with their double talk about their next jobs and destinations. I was sure they were doing this on purpose to impress me so I said that I knew exactly where they were going and that I could not understand why they were making such a secret about it. This amused them greatly and they asked me where I thought they were going. I took a deep breath and said the first thing that came into my head – Yugoslavia. There was a deadly silence: I had guessed right. They whispered to me to shut up and bundled me out of the dining room into someone's bedroom. There I was grilled for over an hour; they would not believe me when I said that I had made it up on the spur of the moment. Their worry was not only that I knew but that the dining room at Shepheard's Hotel was always full of civilians as well as the military, and was reputed to be a hotbed of espionage.

The next morning my friends arrived while I was still in bed, made me dress and marched me off to Military Intelligence where I was interviewed by a series of Intelligence Officers. Eventually they let me go. I learnt afterwards that the only reason I escaped their clutches was that I was due back the next day with my unit – in the middle of the desert. Innocent though I was, Vivian had orders not to let me out of his sight until I was safely on the plane. At the time I knew nothing of this and thought how nice they were all being, taking me to the airport and waiting with me until I left.

The plane back to the desert was another DC. It was as crowded as the flight down. A stuffy old General took me into the Officers' Mess at el Adem – he had probably been told to keep an eye on me, as I was quite capable of finding my own way. We arrived at Tripoli too late for me to find any transport back to the hospital so I spent the night in the Del Mahari Hotel.

The next morning an ammunition ship blew up in the harbour opposite the Hotel. I happened to be in the garden at the time and bits and pieces of glass, concrete and metal flew about in all directions. The harbour was full of ships which hastily got up steam and moved away, but they were not all quick enough and another ammunition ship went up and a tanker caught fire. There was havoc as metal flew about, including shells, which killed two men in the street. A huge piece of metal landed near me so I went inside and continued watching from the windows. No one seemed to know whether it was sabotage or not. Fire engines, fire ships and Military Police were everywhere. David Rowlands arrived and took me back to the hospital.

6

RETURN TO TUNISIA

On 4 September we received orders to leave on the eighth to return to Tunisia. We packed the hospital up and left in the early morning. We drove up the same road for the third time, on our own this time without the rest of the division. We stopped for the first night at a small village called Altremenia and heard to our delight that Italy had surrendered to the Allies.

The following day we arrived at our new site. We set up our hospital on farmland a few miles from the small town of Grombalia. From a small road a farm track led to a green stubble field on the side of a slope in a valley surrounded by hills with a small gap in the hills which gave us a view to the sea. We pitched our tents near a small spinney of fir trees. The slope where we were was quite steep so that we had to remember to leave our cars in gear, facing downhill and their wheels blocked with stones. It was much cooler there than in Tripolitania with a soft wind blowing. The hospital was about twenty miles from the rest of the division with meant a lot of driving for us to keep in touch with the post, transmissions, HQ and so on.

We could buy fruit and vegetables in Grombalia village, which was on the road to Tunis. It was inhabited entirely by Arabs and on market days they were picturesque, the men wearing bright turbans and coloured sashes round their robes and the Berber women in brightly coloured dresses with scarves around their heads.

Very soon several of our friends from the First Armoured Division arrived to welcome us. The Colonel was not amused, and stamped off saying: 'Ze English are worse than ze flies'. The farmer who owned the land was reputed to be a Vichyist and to have given hospitality to Rommel and his Generals, so the Colonel had no hesitation in bullying him into putting three bedrooms and the use of a bathroom at the disposal of the officers. We drew lots for the rooms; Jocelyn won one and the French officers had the other two.

The following days we all had a lot of driving to do. I also worked sometimes in the hospital wards, taking the place of the sisters when they had days off or went on leave. The war seemed far away; when we were not on duty we had a round of parties with the faithful division of 'Rhinos' of the First armoured division and Eighth armoured brigade and the First Guards brigade which had come out with the First Army when they landed in Algeria.

In November the rains came and very soon the farm track and field began to get churned up by the trucks and ambulances. With the rains it became quite cold and all the tents leaked. Our wet clothes and bedding became difficult to dry out and the hospital orderlies had great difficulty drying sheets and towels.

While the division trained its new recruits under the command of General Brosset and re-equipped with most American material, we continued to nurse the medical and accident cases of the division. In all we drew nearly 10,000 extra rations in 80 days, which shows that we were, as usual, full and busy.

The Senegalese saved all their pay to have their beautiful white teeth pulled out and replaced with gold ones. With a full mouth of gold teeth they would eventually return to their village, rich and successful warriors, and would be highly regarded for the remainder of their lives with their wealth for all to see and admire. Although they worked so hard they were good tempered, kind and happy men, laughing and joking all day long and with the simplicity of children. We became very fond of them.

There were several regiments of tirailleurs in the division, in fact they made up most of the infantry. They proved brave and fearless soldiers, wonderful patients when wounded, hardly ever complaining even when their dressings were renewed, however painful. The only time their morale was affected was if a limb had to be amputated because if they lost as much as a finger they would return to their village as an outcast instead of a hero. According to their belief it was a disgrace to lose any part of their bodies and difficult, if not impossible, to enter their heaven. Often, when they were discharged from hospital, they would commit suicide rather than return home.

In contrast, they were very bad medical patients for they had little knowledge of, or faith in western medicine; once away from their medicine men and witch doctors, they would give up the fight, dying from pneumonia, dysentery or some other illness in spite of modern medicine and sulphanilamides. They were also quite capable of dying literally of fright. One day I was helping the Colonel in the operating theatre, putting a plaster cast jacket on a Tirailleur who had fallen out of a lorry and badly damaged a vertebra in his back. The Colonel had not explained what he intended to do before he anaesthetised the patient, so when he came round from the anaesthetic and discovered he could not move he stopped breathing – we had to give him artificial respiration while we removed the plaster. The Colonel showed him the empty jacket, put it on an orderly to show how it worked, and explained why he had used it. The man was then re-anaesthetised and put into a new jacket; when he came round he was all smiles and delighted with his new uniform.

Our two personal Senegalese orderlies, Bellou and Jean, were charming and looked after us with much devotion, almost as if they were children. They used to bring us little presents and photographs of themselves and spare parts for our cars, which they had found in the desert. We knew all their family histories – who was married, how many children they had, their ambitions and their fears. They guarded us from uninvited guests, inquisitive Italians and scavenging Arabs.

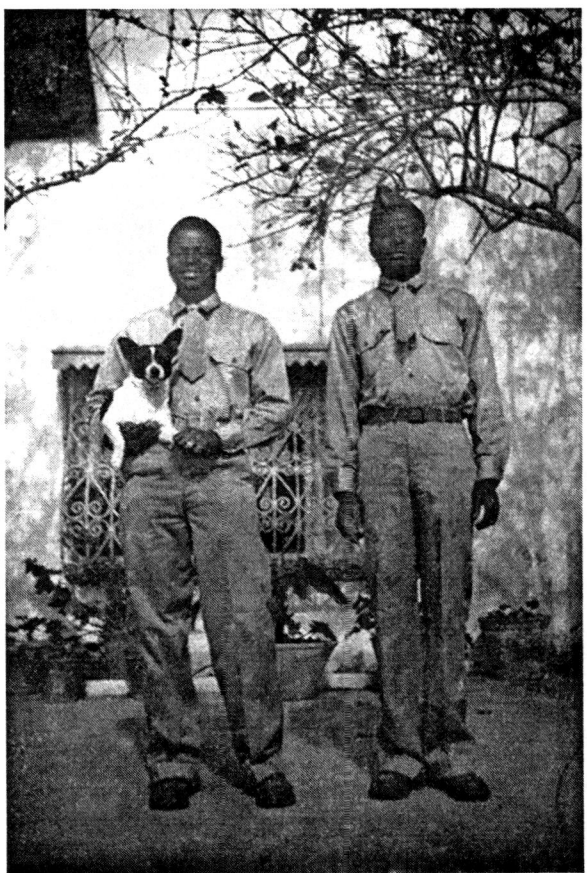

Our orderlies with Whisky the pie-dog.

At the end of November, Biddy and I were sent to Algiers to collect medical equipment and take our almoner, Lieutenant Aurès who, now that Algeria had been liberated, requested a transfer. He was replaced by Lieutenant Duprez who remained with us until the end of the war. We set off with Aurès in my car (82) at an early hour, and drove over the Atlas mountains through Le Kef, Souk Ahras and Constantine. The scenery was magnificent with long empty stretches of uninhabited countryside. Every few yards there was a hairpin bend, some so sharp that we had to reverse to get round them. Biddy, for the first time in her life, felt car sick. A slippery road, due to torrential rain, slowed down our progress. We hoped to reach Setif by nightfall but did not make it due to bad weather and our lights short-circuiting when we switched them on. We were lucky to find a small village which boasted a garage whose owner let us spend the night. Aurès slept on a camp bed provided by the proprietor, while Biddy and I slept in the car. It was freezing cold as we had no blankets, but better than being outside in the rain. Luckily we had plenty of whisky and bully beef and the garage owner brought us hot water the next morning so we could wash our faces and make some Nescafé. We were unable to repair the lights so couldn't leave until daybreak.

We eventually arrived in Algiers early the next afternoon, bedraggled and tired after an unpleasant drive through mist and fog. We deposited Aurès at the French Lycée in the centre of town and then booked ourselves into the Victoria Hotel, which was nothing better than a transit hotel – very scruffy, but we did manage to get a bedroom with wash basins. After cleaning up we had our first proper meal for 36 hours.

Next morning we picked our car up from the garage, checked the electrical system, and serviced the car ourselves in the garage. We had time to do some shopping and window gazing and sent two boxes of oranges home to our families. (They took so long to arrive that there was nothing left except small bits of dried-up rind.) I then went down to the docks in the car to collect our medical equipment while Biddy went to have our travel permits stamped and signed.

We completed our mission by lunch time but, as we were not due to leave until the following morning, we contacted the Queen's Bays, who were stationed near Blida, and spent the rest of the day with them before taking the coast road back to Tunisia and the hospital next day. It was a never-to-be-forgotten drive through awe-inspiring scenic beauty alternating between tortuous roads winding their way up and down precipices with sheer drops to the sea below, through tunnels with signs saying: 'Beware of falling rocks', round more hairpin bends and through cork forests which opened into green pastures. Beyond Djid the country suddenly changed, the mountains were left behind and we descended into open plains, marsh lands, rivers and streams, bridges and fields. There were large flocks of sheep and goats, herds of cattle and horses. In one small valley we passed groups of Arabs hurrying along the road until they reached a narrow track winding its way up the side of a hill; we could see a trail of people resembling ants continuing for miles up the hillside, but never found out where they were going.

During our drive we saw monkeys in the cork forest, the first I had seen in Africa, and round a bend a mongoose crossed our road. We arrived at Philippeville as it was getting dark and found a garage for the car. The YWCA gave us a cup of tea and offered to put us up for the night on mattresses. We wandered round Philippeville for an hour but there was not much to see. It was a dreary French colonial town with a large harbour. Back at the YWCA we had a good supper and, when the dining room had been cleared, two mattresses were brought in and we settled down for the night.

As soon as it was light we collected the car and, after a cup of tea, set off again. It was raining hard so our progress was slow. We drove through Le Monapes, a fairly large Arab town, and bypassed Bone. It was a bad road, full of bumps and pot-holes, later climbing into the mountains again. We descended after a few miles and reached the sea. We travelled through the fishing village of La Calle and away from the coast again through Tabarka and Béja where we joined the road to Tunis and Medjez, arriving back at the hospital at three o'clock. It had been an exciting trip and a welcome break.

By the beginning of December the weather conditions had deteriorated further and the entire hospital encampment had become a sodden morass of mud and damp. Moving around became more and more difficult for personnel and vehicles and it became impossible to keep anything or anyone dry for long. The patients suffered the most, with drips of rain falling on them from leaks in the tents and damp rising from the earth on which their beds stood. It became so bad that the Colonel looked around for more solid housing. Eventually he found what he was searching for at Hammamet, a charming holiday village with luxurious villas with gardens reaching down to the sea. The old Arab town is on the other side of the bay and a fort looks out over the sea. At first, General Brosset said the hospital was not to move but he finally agreed; the hospital wards were housed in the Hotel du Golfe with supplementary tents alongside. The Colonel installed himself in a small villa between the hotel and the sea and the rest of the personnel were housed in villas around the hotel. We women were given a delightful villa – the Villa Plumbago – which had a large garden of the blue shrubs which, to our delight, were in bloom all the time we were there. I was particularly lucky to find a small room on the ground floor which no one else wanted. It had its own front door opening into the garden and another locked door, which I naturally broke open. I discovered a bathroom stacked from floor to ceiling with flower vases, urns and dozens of mirrors of all shapes and sizes. I managed to clear enough away to be able to use the bath. I found the cold water tap was in running order, which was a surprise, and so I had a suite to myself.

This was the first time we had had a roof over our heads since we were at Buseilli in Egypt and we certainly appreciated the return to civilisation. We would have enjoyed meeting the owner of the villa who obviously had a penchant for mirrors for they were everywhere and very beautiful, but he had fled before the Germans arrived. The villa still had a few pieces of furniture left; we spent days cleaning it up and putting it in order. We collected driftwood for the large fireplace in the salon and 'borrowed' electric light bulbs and other necessities from the surrounding empty villas. When we had completed our work we gave several parties to the unit and the division. While we were there we made the acquaintance of several of the local inhabitants who had defied the Germans and Italians and stayed on.

One of the kindest to me were an octogenarian couple called Ormond. They lived in a large house – the Villa Ormond – on the edge of the Arab quarter. Madame Ormond was American, the sister of Sargent, the artist, and the house was full of his paintings. Monsieur Ormond was Swiss and they had taken the precaution of running up the Swiss flag when the Nazis arrived, which saved them from being molested and their house pillaged. They invited me to several meals which were always delicious and generally ended with champagne and brandy. They told me many stories of the German occupation – not always pleasant. Through them I became friends with Violet Henson who lived in the Villa Henson in the rich European side of Hammamet. She was English, married to an American who the Germans had carted off and put in a civilian prison camp in France. Her house had been ransacked by both the Germans and Italians, her furniture broken up for firewood, her fine library of books stolen and tanks driven through her once beautiful garden. She lent me the few books that remained and told me fascinating stories of some of the rich absent landlords. She was having a very difficult time. She had no news of her husband, no money to pay her servants or to buy food and hardly any clothes – they had been taken by the Italians – and her house was in a shambles. We tried to help Violet but there was not much we could do beyond slipping her army rations and the odd army shirt and jersey. When we left Hammamet I gave her my two pet rabbits which, I learned later, had multiplied and provided her with the odd meal.

Air Chief Marshall Cunningham, an Australian, was living at that time at the Villa Sebastian, where Churchill had spent some of his convalescence when recovering from the attack of pneumonia he had contracted at the summit meeting with President Roosevelt in Algiers. Several army chiefs had cast envious eyes at the villa as it was the most fabulous house. The entire décor was in black and white down to the rugs on the floors and the bindings of the books on the shelves. Miraculously it had not been pillaged or damaged in any way; the owner was an Argentinean and reputed to be pro-Nazi. The villa was built around an inner courtyard which was designed as a Roman bath with pillars surrounding a sunken bath and the entire roof was of Lalique glass. More Roman pillars led from a garden door down to a large swimming pool at the bottom of the garden which overlooked the sea and sandy beach. Upstairs was a single bedroom and bathroom where, we were told, the third Madame Sebastian, a rich American lady, was banished while Monsieur Sebastian entertained Arab boys in his downstairs bedroom suite.

We were invited us to several parties at the villa and we always enjoyed going there and imagined what it must have been like in pre-war times. Signed photographs of famous people – including one of the Duke of Windsor – were scattered around the reception rooms.

Christmas and New Year were both celebrated in true Anglo–French fashion – carol singing by the FAU on Christmas Eve, followed by midnight mass and French Christmas supper. English lunch on Christmas Day of roast pork, no turkey alas, but the NAAFI supplied a Christmas pudding which the French said they enjoyed as much as we did. In the evening the Quakers presented a concert, with topical sketches and original verse and more to eat and drink. The French took over on New Year's Eve with another party to which General de Larminat, General Brosset and all the Colonels of the divisional regiments came. The mess was decorated with brilliant posters by Yantze our radiologist. There was more acting and sketches and Germaine Sablon sang, but the highlight of the evening was the Colonel singing his own words to *Madame la Marquise.*

7

ON TO ITALY

In our cosy house of bricks and mortar, complete with garden, we quickly collected a variety of animals: lost kittens, a curious squirrel-like animal – which, alas, died when we fed it on the wrong food – and a pair of rabbits, a white one with blue eyes, given to me by Thibaux for Christmas, and a black and white one which had adopted Biddy and me when we were sharing a tent at Grombalia. I saw it sitting in the space between our beds one morning and fearing that I had DTs I quickly shut my eyes again and waited for Biddy to wake up. Luckily for me the rabbit was real and, as it showed no sign of leaving, we built it a hutch, where it lived happily. When we moved to Hammamet it was given the freedom of a disused dog kennel, complete with wired-in run and was joined at Christmas by the white one.

A small black and white pie-dog adopted me at Hammamet. I called him 'Whisky' and he soon grew fat on bully beef. He followed me everywhere and was very possessive, nipping visitors' legs if he got a chance. I could not take him with me when we left Hammamet but I found him a good home with a farmer's wife.

The weather continued to be cold and wet, with violent winds and thunderstorms, and we considered ourselves very lucky to be under a roof. Our days were fully occupied driving the officers around and being sent on missions.

By 1 April 1943 the weather had become warm and sunny again and we played our annual football match against the officers of the hospital. Most of the division turned out to watch and de Larminat came too. We always had help from one or two Quakers dressed up as women. The Colonel and the officers handicapped themselves by wearing fancy dress and putting a leg and arm or two in plaster or splints. That year there was quite a gale blowing which took the ball down one side and out. The umpires made certain we won by giving 'off side' if the ball came near our goal.

At Grombalia and at Hammamet I worked frequently in the hospital, relieving a sister whenever she had a day off or leave. I had hospital training and was State Registered; I was a driver first and foremost but was always willing to help out in the hospital. Naturally when the division went into action and wounded started to arrive I worked full time in the hospital.

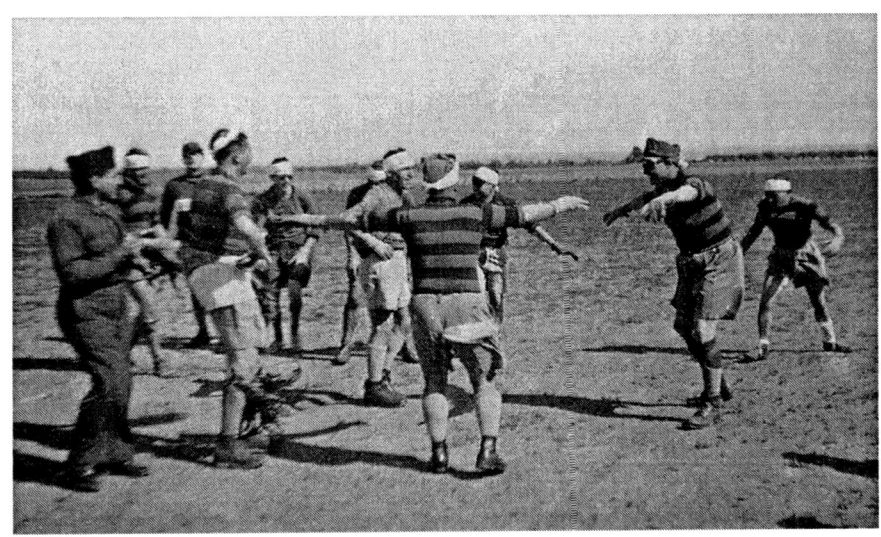

Tunisia 1944 – Spears officers before the annual football
match against the women. The women always won.

At Grombalia and Hammamet we had one day off a week as well as other free time when we were either 'on call', driving or mending our cars which, as they grew older, needed more and more attention. When neither we, nor our own workshop (who were marvellous at getting all the vehicles repaired) could mend them, we took them to the Divisional Atelier Lourd who had all the necessary equipment and would replace engines, gear boxes and so on.

There were only four drivers at this time – Iris, Jocelyn, Biddy and me. Kit was in England with a badly broken finger which could not be looked after by the hospital. We had a lot of driving to do. Jocelyn generally did the post and collecting orders from HQ, which she enjoyed doing as it meant meeting the top brass. We did not mind most of the time.

18 January – The hospital and staff are inspected by General de Lattre and the French Minister for War in de Gaulle's cabinet. We had to dress up in our smart uniform and, like all French Generals, de Lattre was late – an hour and a half. He shook hands with everyone and never said a word. Later he complained that the hospital was dirty because he found some orange peel on the floor. After the parade I changed into my working clothes again and helped Kit decarbonise Marguerite. When that was accomplished I took two new nurses into Naboul where they wandered around and bought material and some of the pottery for Naboul is famous.

Susan Travers joined us for the inspection. She had been a patient in the hospital with dysentery. Susan was Koenig's driver while he was in command of the division and had driven him out of Bir Hakim a few hours before it was overrun by the Germans. His car was pitted with several bullet holes. When Koenig moved on and Brosset took command Susan was adopted by the Foreign Legion, the only woman to ever serve with them. While a patient at the hospital we looked after Josephine, her Alsatian dog. Susan had her hair cut short like a boy's and always wore battle dress, never a skirt. The first time I saw her she was having lunch at our end of the mess table. I thought she was a man and wondered what he was doing at our end. She was always very friendly and after the war we learnt that she married one of the sergeants from the Legion; he was of German origin and they returned to live in England in the New Forest and had two sons.

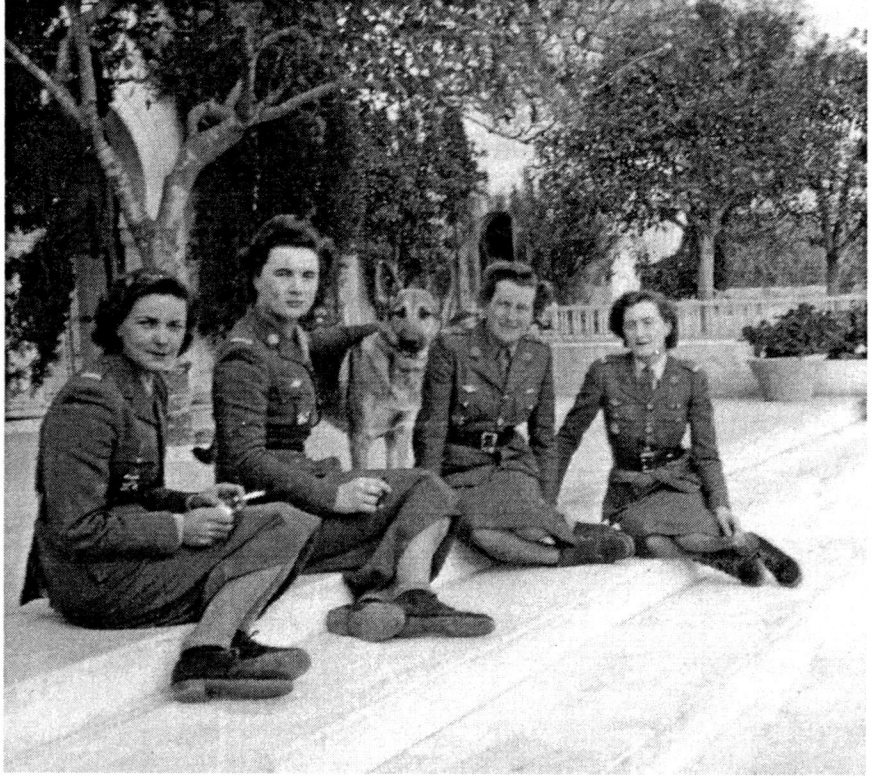

The author, Biddy, Jocelyn and Iris, with Susan Travers' dog Josephine, waiting to be inspected by General de Lattre. They always kept us waiting.

Our army rations at this time in the war were very uncertain. We, and the whole division, were in the process of being handed over to the Americans and neither they nor the British wanted to be bothered with us so Père Boileau had to scrounge what he could. Luckily there was fruit and vegetables and the odd bit of fish and meat to be bought in the markets and I still drew NAAFI rations, which included whisky at 8/- and gin at 6/-, and I was able to continue doing this until we arrived in France.

When we finally sampled the American rations we thought they were marvellous to begin with – white bread, butter, ham and eggs cooked together, and spam. There were packed rations, sufficient for one man for seven days or seven men for one day. They even contained lavatory paper, cigarettes and solid fuel for brewing up. Sadly we soon tired of them. Everything tasted the same – completely tasteless and too much cellophane wrapping. We longed for bully beef again and mousetrap cheese.

While we were at Hammamet four French women were wished upon us. We were not at all pleased, as it was contrary to the statute agreed between General de Gaulle and Lady Spears which laid down that all female personnel were to be English and chosen by her. However the four, who had been sent from London to the division, remained with us. They were originally a blood transfusion unit, but we had our own and no one in the division wanted them. Jobs which did not interfere with either the sisters or the drivers were found for them, and they remained with us until the end of the war.

Germaine Sablon also arrived at the unit but with Lady Spears' blessing. She was given a tent and organised a *foyer* for the patients where they could buy cigarettes, soap, razors and so on. She helped them with their letters and cheered them up.

On 12 April all the patients who were well enough were evacuated to their units. Those who were not went to the large civilian hospital in Tunis, and our hospital prepared itself for its next destination – Naples. We checked our stores and equipment, packed up the lorries and staff cars and gave our civilian friends everything we could not take with us, which included all the animals.

We got up at 5.30am and, after a hurried cup of tea, I finished loading 82 with my belongings and collected my passengers – Pam Spears, Joan Pryke and all their belongings. The Nannies always had masses of bits and pieces. They had breakfast ready cooked for me, which was kind and a surprise. Violet Henson arrived, and some Arabs ready to salvage anything we left behind that might be useful. We left in convoy at 8.30; all went well with 82 until we reached the outskirts of Tunis when she spluttered, coughed and died up every hill. I tried everything to keep her going, cleaned out the petrol pump and carburettor and even drained the petrol tank and refilled it – all to no avail. She finally collapsed up a steep hill and refused to start up again. Pam and Joan were very long-suffering and did not complain.

Maintenance came to my assistance – they always travelled last knowing that there would be lame ducks to rescue. They were also unable to get me going and, after we ate a large lunch together, I was ignominiously towed by John Little from Ferryville to Bizerte. A truck was waiting to take me and the sisters to our billets for the night. We threw everything out of 82 on to the truck and then persuaded John to tow 82 and me to the dockside where I abandoned her to the mercies of the FAU. Biddy came to collect me and we arrived at the hostel in time for supper.

We women were lodged in a scruffy hotel near the docks and all hell was let loose the first night we were there. The lights were turned off at the mains at 10pm and immediately hundreds of bugs fell off the ceilings on to our beds. Pandemonium ensued with everyone groping around with torches and a general exodus to the garden. Next day we organised ourselves more efficiently in various bits of the garden and hung up our mosquito nets.

The Colonel arrived the next afternoon to say that the hospital equipment and transport were to be loaded on to two American Liberty ships, the first of which would take our cars and was due to sail at midnight the following day. But – the Americans did not allow women on their Liberty ships. We would be left behind to follow in a passenger ship which was not due to sail for another seven days. No one was pleased with the news, least of all us drivers, who would be unable to supervise the unloading of our cars. It would mean someone else would drive them away from the docks and it was an unwritten law that no one was allowed to drive the cars except us.

The Colonel had a plan. He proposed that we drivers should all dress up as French soldiers and hide ourselves on board away from the American crew until the ship had sailed. We unanimously agreed to this and spent the following day collecting our soldiers' uniforms and rehearsing our parts.

Lieutenant Duprez, gestionnaire, and the Colonel arrived after lunch. Duprez had an order of the day for the Tirailleurs that, under pain of detention, they were not to explode into laughter when they saw us or to draw attention to us in any way. The Colonel was full of confidence, in spite of the fact that the whole division knew what had been arranged. He said that everything was well in hand and that it was time for us to get ready.

Amid lots of laughter we put on large army boots, rough battle dress and scraped our hair under tin hats. Germaine Sablon, with her collection of make up, made up our faces to look grimy and weather beaten. When we were all ready we piled into two lorries and were driven by Captain Coupigny and one of the Quakers to the quayside where the Colonel hid us behind packing cases. He told us that whatever happened we were not to talk. Coupigny was in charge of us and he would answer for us if any Americans arrived and started to ask questions. He would give us the command to march on board. We waited for what seemed to be ages and then the Colonel arrived to say that it was all up and that we were to return to our hotel. One of the newly arrived French girls, Antoinette Bounden who had been with one of the naval blood transfusion units, had got on board before us without any trouble and proceeded to walk around the deck with her long hair flowing behind her. Inevitably, she had been spotted by one of the American Military Police, who made a great hullabaloo.

We were furious at her stupidity. She had let us all down, including the Colonel and Lotte, who had an unpleasant interview with the American OC. Luckily no one discovered us. The Americans immediately put a sentry on each of the gangways to inspect everyone boarding the ship.

We climbed disconsolately back into our lorries and were driven to our billet where we thankfully got out of the scratchy clothes and scrubbed the greasepaint off our faces. The Colonel returned to say goodbye and told us not to worry as he had managed to get us passages on a fast passenger ship due to sail in four days' time. This should overtake the much slower Liberty ship and we should be in Naples with plenty of time to supervise the off-loading of our staff cars and drive them away.

Only half the hospital had embarked on the first Liberty ship; the rest, including the Quakers, heavy lorries and the remainder of the hospital equipment were to embark on another Liberty ship due to leave in a few days' time.

There was panic that night when it started to rain heavily and we had to pick our way up the garden and into the house carrying our bedding. We all got bitten by the army of bugs. We had been left very few rations and no NAAFI stores so the next morning I borrowed a truck from the Quakers and went down to the NAAFI to see what I could scrounge. They were not very helpful and said I had to have the authority of the British officer in charge of the garrison before they would issue me with anything. This was not difficult but it took time and I had another long wait at the NAAFI before I was able to collect what we needed.

After four days of patient waiting, and no sign of our fast passenger ship, we learned that it was not due for another ten days. This meant there was no hope at all of arriving in Naples in time to off-load our cars. Now we really did have to get cracking and somehow find a way of getting over to Italy.

A conference with Solly who was in charge of everyone left behind did more harm than good. He became extremely pompous and kept on repeating that he was responsible for us and if we disobeyed his orders we would be court martialled. We became very cautious after he said this and took care not to provoke him into giving us a direct order. We (the four drivers) decided among ourselves that we would split into two pairs and each pair would try a different route. We would all leave at the same time and go our different ways. The only person we told our plans to was Michael Rowntree, head of the Quakers, and we swore him to secrecy, just in case there was a hue and cry when our disappearance became known. Biddy and Iris made up one pair, Jocelyn and I the other. We took one knapsack between us containing essentials such as toothbrushes and a change of shirt and underclothes.

We left immediately after breakfast, praying that our disappearance would not be noticed until the evening, by which time we expected to be out of Tunisia. Jocelyn and I started off well and succeeded in borrowing an American staff car and driver to take us to the US airforce base at Wyla. Alas, we drew a blank there. The Americans, usually happy-go-lucky about air travel, would not touch us. There had been a hullabaloo concerning two Queen Alexandra army sisters who had hopped a lift to Cairo and found themselves in Crete instead and, together with the crew, were all put in the bag by the occupying Germans. We were, however, able to persuade the sympathetic American driver to take us to the RAF airbase near Tunis and dump us there.

We made a very inauspicious start with the adjutant in charge of flying. He was not at all impressed by our sad story of our old cars being unloaded without our assistance. He told us that we must have a written authority from Military HQ in Algiers before he would allow us on any of his planes. This was clearly impossible, as he well knew, so I just launched into a long diatribe against the ridiculous amount of red tape which bogged down everything in the army. I had no idea that this happened to be his favourite hobby horse. It had a lightning effect. In a matter of seconds he had issued us with all the necessary bits of bumph, including 'priority two' travel permits, and two transit vouchers for the night at the Majestic Hotel in Tunis. He lent us a staff car to take us there and invited us to dine with him that evening at the hotel. He was a strange little man; he had only one eye and it was impossible to tell if he was looking at you.

As soon as we reached the Majestic we wrote a letter to Mike telling him of our good fortune and then enjoyed the luxury of a hot bath, our first since October. Layers of dirt peeled off us; I had to have two lots of water before I felt really clean.

Dinner with our benefactor, Squadron Leader Barrington (whom we never saw or heard of again), began pleasantly until, out of the blue, General Brosset appeared. We were drinking our soup and nearly choked over it when we saw him. We tried to hide our faces and hoped that he would not recognise us, but of course he did. He beckoned me over to his table and asked me what we were doing in Tunis. I had no alternative but to tell him the truth, all except the bit about disobeying Solly. To my relief he was highly delighted with our initiative and even offered to help Biddy and Iris if they had not succeeded on their own. We prayed that we and they would have left Tunisia before he contacted Solly.

A violent thunderstorm during the night made it impossible to sleep and we wondered what condition the airfield would be in next morning. We were called at 6.30am by an orderly with a cup of tea and taken to the airfield in the Squadron Leader's staff car. Everywhere was flooded. As we had feared, all planes were grounded and all incoming planes diverted. We were told that they hoped our plane would get off eventually if there was no further rain. Our knapsacks were loaded on to the plane and ourselves on to a lorry, which splashed its way along the runway to the plane. Then we were told 'No flights to Italy today' and had to collect our knapsacks and return to the hotel.

Desperate at the thought that Solly would have learnt from General Brosset our whereabouts and would get us back, I pleaded with the American pilot. I painted a lurid picture of us in prison and our cars falling from the cranes into the sea. He finally agreed to think about it in an hour or two.

We were able to get breakfast of a sort at the airport canteen and after a long wait were put into the lorry again and this time loaded on to the plane. We roared down the runway through a foot of water and succeeded in taking off at the very last yard. Visibility was almost nil to begin with but improved after a while. We flew over Lampadusa, Sicily, and the coast of Corsica; then turned inland over Italy and eastwards over the mountains to land at Bari. While the plane refuelled we had a quick lunch and flew on to Foggia where we had another stop. We had a very bumpy flight to Naples. I noticed a RAF officer sitting opposite me becoming greener and greener. I asked him if he felt airsick. He whispered 'No' but added that we were flying much too low and that one air pocket would take us into the side of the mountain. We had been quite happy until then, blissfully unaware of any danger. I watched Jocelyn, who watched me, and we both ended up the same colour as the RAF officer. However, all was well. Our pilot even gave us a good look at Vesuvius, quietly smouldering, by flying around and over the crater.

Southern Italy looked, from the air, very like Tunisia – the same olive groves and vineyards. The towns and villages appeared to be built on the hilltops instead of in the valleys. There were church spires and cobbled roofs. We saw no large houses or farms, no hedges or fences. The olive groves were occasionally surrounded by stone walls or ditches. Strange little squat hummocks, resembling large beehives, were dotted about in all the groves. We wondered whether they were for human habitation or for animals. We flew over several rivers and streams of various widths, none containing more than a trickle of water. We saw a few flocks of sheep and herds of cows. Every inch of the land appeared to be cultivated right up to the hillsides and barren peaks. Some of the hillsides were wooded with spruce or fir, but it was difficult to make out from the air. At last we landed safely, and thankfully, at Naples airport.

An army truck was waiting to take all the passengers into Naples, and dropped Jocelyn and me off at the British officers' transit hotel in the centre of the town, a rather grubby and battered building called the Patria. To our surprise and delight Biddy and Iris were already installed there. We immediately exchanged accounts of our adventures – theirs seemed to be much more enterprising than ours. Iris had hitch-hiked a lift to the airstrip outside Bizerte and found there was a good chance of them hopping a lift the next day on a RAF freight plane. She and Biddy returned to the hostel where no one seemed to have noticed our absence. Early next morning they tiptoed through the sleeping Nannies and made their way on foot to the airstrip which was quite a distance. At midday they were smuggled on to a freight plane, sitting uncomfortably on and between packing cases. Their flight was direct to Naples and they arrived an hour before we did.

So there we were in Naples awaiting the arrival of the Liberty ship which was not due for another two days. Biddy made contact with Tommy Rivers Bulkeley of the Scots Guards, who was attached to his brigade's HQ somewhere beyond Naples. Bobby Petre drove us there for dinner in a very uncomfortable jeep, refusing to share a rubber ring he sat on to lessen the bumps. Biddy and Tommy decided that evening to get married before our division went into action. I rushed round Naples trying to collect all the necessary permissions and papers for them – luckily the British Town Major was a friend of my parents and through him I got all the necessary bumph. They were married the next day at Tommy's HQ with a pipe major to pipe them away – and champagne appeared from somewhere. Iris and I attended the wedding. Biddy and Tommy were unable to have a honeymoon until much later as Biddy had to justify her disobedience to Solly by off-loading her car.

We spent most of 27 April travelling to and from the docks waiting for the *SS Adams*. She finally docked at 4.30pm. Only the Colonel was allowed off the ship. We were there to greet him as he came down the gangway and he was amazed to see us there. The personnel left on board shouted down to us that they were very hungry and thirsty, so we tore around trying to find them something. Most of the shops were shut and those remaining open had very little to sell. Captain St Hilier, General Brosset's Chief of Staff, turned up and said he could spare some wine from the HQ. We took that and some oranges we found in the market to them. The ship was not to be unloaded until the following day, so we returned to the Patria for the night.

28 April – After hanging about all day at the docks our cars were eventually unloaded at 7pm when it was almost dark and, in spite of all our precautions, my poor old 82 was dropped on her nose on the quayside and her radiator smashed. By 11.30pm all the vehicles were off the ship and lined up in convoy and we started off in the dark with, as usual, no lights permitted. I was at the end of a tow rope. Tommy Bulkeley had come along to help and drove 91 for us as we were short of one driver. The Colonel led the convoy as Mike Rowntree was still in Bizerte. We reached our destination, Albanova, a small, dusty and dirty village some 30 miles from Naples, at 1am. We parked the cars and lorries in a courtyard with guards to keep watch over them and returned to the Patria in Iris's 64 for what was left of the night.

29 April – It took me a long time to get a permit to have 82's radiator mended at a Rome REME workshop; for good measure, I asked for a new engine as well. We then collected our knapsacks from the Patria and set off for Albanova, which looked completely different in daylight and not so dismal. It was a picturesque road lined with trees with vines growing between them, festooned in loops from one tree to the next. Albanova itself was a very poor and primitive village with small peasant houses nestling beside a few farms of grey stone each side of the one main street of beaten earth, with an open drain for sewage running down along each side. When the wind blew, or any vehicle drove past, dust far dirtier than the desert sand rose in fine particles, covering everything. There were no shops; the church and school were the only municipal buildings.

The little village was overcrowded with refugee children and orphans from a bombed-out school in Naples. They were looked after by the nuns from a neighbouring convent. At every door and window women and children peeped out fearfully, wondering, I suppose, how they would fare at the hands of these newly arrived French soldiers.

Apart from our military vehicles the only traffic was bullock carts each pulled by beautiful white oxen with large gentle brown eyes, their heads bent under a wooden yoke.

The children soon lost their fear and followed us in droves, begging for sweets and cigarettes. They were very unattractive, clothed in rags, with snotty noses and covered in sores from scabies and lice. They begged with whining voices and snatched our offerings from our hands, running away quickly to squabble over their booty. They stole whenever they had the chance.

Our officers were billeted in a house near the church and we drivers (and the sisters when they arrived), were lodged in one large room in a farmhouse which boasted the only water closet in the village. This was situated at the end of an open balcony, a very primitive affair with buckets of water to flush the pan, but an improvement on the hole in the ground. The officers' mess was in our house and the square courtyard of the farm made a good garage for our cars. We were kept busy in the days that followed, driving the officers around. One day I drove the Colonel to where our camp would be placed when the division made its attack across the Garigliano River, about fifty miles from Albanova towards Cassino and four miles from the front line. The Colonel chose a site on a hillside between the small towns of St Georgia and Conea.

One day, while we were at Albanova and in the middle of our lunch, the village curé arrived in a great state to ask the Colonel for his help in saving the life of a baby which had fallen into its mother's washing tub. The Colonel told me to come with him and we ran down the street to a hovel. We fought our way through a crowd of wailing women and found the baby lying on a dirty piece of blanket on the floor. He was completely blue and moribund and not breathing. The Colonel immediately started artificial respiration while I got the women to heat pans of water and fill empty wine bottles with boiling water. I then wrapped them in rags and put them all around the baby, who continued to be icy cold and lifeless. After what seemed to be ages the baby suddenly took a shallow breath and we could at last feel his pulse, weak and ragged. The Colonel then left and told me to stay until I was satisfied that the baby was out of danger. After a few minutes the baby gave a weak cry, whereupon all the women crowded in, leaving the baby no space to breathe. In desperation I picked the baby up and carried him into the little courtyard, telling the mother to keep the door shut and only let in the relay of women reheating the bottles. It was nearly an hour before the colour returned to the baby's ashen face and body and he began to move his limbs and lift up his head. I gave him some warm milk and brandy from a teaspoon and left him with his mother.

I had never heard women wailing like that before. They sounded like a lot of banshees and it was frightening. When it was clear the baby had recovered they started crying that it was a miracle and the wailing began all over again.

The Sisters and Quakers who had been left behind with Solly in Bizerte arrived on 2 May with the remainder of the hospital equipment. They told us that one of the Sisters, Betty Corthay, and one of the French girls, Yvonne le Motte had left the hostel in Bizerte, following our example. Unlike us they had not arrived and no one knew where they were or what had happened to them. The Colonel was furious and had to report their disappearance to HQ who had no alternative but to send out alerts and to start a search for them. After a week had passed with no news of them they both turned up together. They had smuggled themselves aboard a Liberty ship dressed as men and hidden in one of the holds for the six-day voyage. They had lived on the dry rations they had taken with them and had had a most uncomfortable trip. It was an idiotic escapade as, unlike us, they had absolutely no reason to leave the others – no cars to off-load, no driving to do – and they knew perfectly well that the hospital could neither move nor open until they and the rest of the equipment was reassembled. As a result of their escapade Betty was sacked and Yvonne (who could not be returned to France) was exchanged for Sister Kelsey from the Ambulance Chirurgicale Légère – a bonus for us. Kelsey was a highly trained and efficient nurse and had originally joined the Free French when they were fighting in Eritrea. The disobedience of these two boomeranged on to us and we had to be punished as well with fifteen days' CB. This did not prevent us from driving our cars but we were forbidden to leave the camp, except on duty, or to receive visits in our tents, except from our own officers. It turned out that we were so busy in the hospital by this time that there was no question of any off duty.

lère Division Française Libre
DIRECTION DU SERVICE DE STE
№ 3459/D

P U N I T I O N
-o-o-o-o-o-o-

Par ordre du Médécin Lieutenant Colonel LOTTE, Directeur du Service

de Santé de la 1ère D.F.L.

une punition de 15 jours d'arrêts de rigueur est infligée aux

Conductrices :

Miss PATTINSON BIDDY (Mrs Berkeley)
Miss HOWELL EVANS
Mrs RUSSELL
Miss GOODWIN

MOTIF: Désobéissance caractérisée à un ordre donné par le Médécin
Lieutenant officiellement chargé de representer le Médécin
Chef dans le détachement dont elles faisaient partie.-

Le 7 Mai 1944
Le Médécin Lieutenant-Colonel LOTTE
Directeur du Sce de Santé de la 1è DFL

Signé: LOTTE

COPIE CERTIFIEE CONFORME:

S.P.82070,le 10 Mai 1944
Le Médécin Lieutenant Colonel VERNIER, Médécin
Chef de l'AMBULANCE HADFIELD SPEARS,

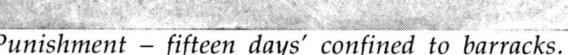

Punishment – fifteen days' confined to barracks.

8

ACROSS THE GARIGLIANO RIVER

Immediately the unit was reunited we started packing up for active service again. The staff cars with their load of sisters left on the afternoon of 4 May and the remainder of the hospital in convoy during the night.

The layout of the hospital was planned the following day and the tent positions pegged out. We chose a good site for our own tents, on the edge of a hill overlooking a valley with an uninterrupted view of the hills beyond. The Colonel gave us all a pep talk confirming that a big attack against the German lines on the Garigliano river was due to start in three or four days' time. No tents were to be erected until it began as our arrival, and that of the division, had to be kept secret. We all slept in or around our vehicles and it was lucky for everyone that the weather was warm and dry.

Kit returned to us on 7 May having had great difficulty in getting out of England due to the impending Overlord invasion of France. No communications or people were being allowed out of the fortress island for security reasons. Kit's story of how she managed it is a saga on its own.

Shortly before the attack General Brosset sent out an order that we were to wear our tin hats whenever driving to a forward area. As we were already in one, this meant all the time. We kept them under the driving seats of our cars, but I don't think any of us ever remembered to wear them. I got a rocket from General Brosset one day for not wearing mine. He passed me driving at great speed and, in spite of the cloud of dust his jeep raised, he recognised me, turned round and rushed after me. When he had stopped shouting at me I pointed out that he wasn't wearing one either. He said that was different and made me put mine on.

Iris and I went off to Naples taking Pam and Arnold Spiers, who hoped to get married before the attack began. Iris wanted to have her car's almost non-existent brakes relined and I wanted to collect the unit's post and our weekly NAAFI supply. I managed to get a whole set of maps of the forward area, which was very useful, a quantity of collapsible chairs and tin mugs for the mess and a battery lamp for myself. It was getting dark by the time I had finished all my errands and set off for the hospital again. When I reached Alberta, 82 began to cough and splutter and finally died on me halfway up a hill. I took down the petrol pump and carburettor and cleaned them both but she still would not start so I tried the last desperate and dangerous trick I knew of, which was sucking the petrol up the pipe, but to no avail. A black American soldier stopped and offered help but he was no mechanic. Finally, a British breakdown lorry drove by and offered to take me as far as Capua. At Capua another truck agreed, after some persuasion, to tow me the rest of the way to the hospital. I did not enjoy the experience of bumping along in the dark with no lights, and clouds of dust obscuring the brake light of the truck towing me. I was thankful to arrive at the hospital with 82 and myself in one piece. I gratefully gave the driver some beer and food before he set off again.

Great activity was taking place in the dark on my return and I learnt that General Alexander had issued an order that the long-awaited attack across the Garigliano river was to begin at midnight – with the Free French positioned between the Eighth Army on the right and the American Fifth Army, under General Clark, on the left.

We all helped to put up the big yellow tents; between them, they housed 160 beds which we made up in complete darkness before laying out the instruments and dressings in the surgical wards. The resuscitation ward was put between the X-ray tent and the theatres.

At the stroke of midnight the big guns sited all around us opened up. The noise was terrific; no one slept through the barrage. Howitzers, 88s, and 105 mm tracer bullets and flares illuminated the sky. The gunfire reverberated around the hills so that the boom and crash, whistle and bang merged into an orchestration of sounds accompanying a giant firework display, with death in the audience. It was so deafening that it was impossible to distinguish between sending and receiving. Happily, this first night, only a few duds, which did not explode, fell around the hospital.

At 3am the first ambulances of wounded arrived and continued in an ever-increasing stream. At daybreak I tried to get 82 working again with the help of Biddy and Kit. We removed the petrol tank and pipes and cleaned out the entire petrol system – the tank was filthy and full of water, which certainly contributed to my troubles.

By midday the hospital wards were almost full and I changed my role from driver to nurse and relieved Margaret, who had been working without a break in the resuscitation tent. We decided to work eight-hour shifts until the rush was over. Work in the resuscitation ward meant inspecting each ambulance load of stretchers as they were laid out in rows outside the tent and deciding which of the wounded needed either blood or plasma the most urgently. Abdominal wounds were always top priority as they had to be operated upon within twelve hours if the patient was to have any chance of recovery. Any further delay and peritonitis would set in; even with the miraculous sulphanilamide drugs, the prognosis was poor. Very often there were as many as twelve or more perforations, each to be found and stitched up.

Amputations and wounds which caused great loss of blood were our other priority. Getting a transfusion working in time was often the difference between life and death, and more difficult in the dark with only a torch to see by. We had room for only four stretchers in our tent; having transfused the patients we sent them straight into one of the two adjacent operating theatres. The Colonel worked in one and Capitaine Thibaux in the other – it was like a conveyor belt. Sometimes we had to fix up extra transfusions outside the tent among the stretchers lying on the ground. When the rush was very great, we pushed spare tent poles into the ground to hang the bottles from.

When we reached Italy all our medical supplies were American and, in many ways, superior to the British and much more extravagant. Syringes, needles and tubing were all separately packed and individually sterilised, made to be used once and then thrown away. But, and it was a very big but, each item was sealed under pressure in a tin which had a key attached to it and made to open like a sardine tin. Unfortunately they often broke off halfway round and we cut and bruised our fingers trying to open them in a hurry. Having finally opened a tin, we then had to tear open tough plastic wrappings and assemble the pieces of tubing, glass connections and needles. The plasma came in two sealed jars: one of saline water, the other of plasma crystals. The saline had to be siphoned into the crystals and shaken up – all very time-consuming when a man's life was at stake and seconds counted. Eventually we were given two Senegalese orderlies who did nothing but open tins for us.

The following morning after finishing my eight-hour stint I finished putting the petrol tank and pipes back into my car but she still would not go. I then discovered that her distributor was cracked which meant a journey to the Atelier Lourd to beg another. Having fixed it I went to bed and tried to sleep through the noise of the guns until I was back on the resuscitation ward again.

The wounded lay on stretchers on the ground outside the resuscitation tent. They had labels around their necks or tied to their chests describing the seriousness of their injuries. It was very difficult to read in the dark with the dim torch what their injuries were and it was our one dread that we would miss an urgent case and be responsible for a man's death. If we did we never knew.

Two men died while I was trying to save them. One was a légionnaire who had most of his thigh blown off. He had lost so much blood, in spite of a tight tourniquet, that I could not get blood back into him quickly enough. The other was an American with most of his brain hanging out of his skull so that he could not possibly have survived.

It was a hectic time for everyone. The drivers tried to keep a steady rota of cars on the road to ferry blood and plasma and collect and deliver orders and messages. Sometimes our supply of blood ran out completely. We would then tap the hospital staff or volunteers who were universal blood groups and, when they had given their quota, the staff cars were sent out to collect more from any source they could find.

18 May – A forward unit was dispatched with Captain Thibaux in charge to the front line, which had now advanced 15 miles from us. This left the Colonel as the only surgeon with the hospital proper, but it also meant that the most urgent cases would be treated before they reached us. That night was not nearly so hectic in our little tent and for the first time I was able to tidy it up a bit.

The following evening the Colonel announced at supper that the hospital was to close down at 8pm and that we were to move up to the front line again in two days' time, near the town of St Georgia. Evacuating our 200 patients, taking down tents and packing everything took a whole day. The next morning I drove Père Boileau to Caserta and Alabnora where he bought meat and vegetables from the Italians. He gave me a present of two eggs – I wrote it in my diary, so they must have been a rare treat. When I got back I helped take down our own tents and then packed my possessions and those of my two passengers, Joan and Margaret, into 82. It started to rain at teatime, so we decided to spend the night in the car, not much room and very uncomfortable. I was in the front seat, and kept falling off; I woke up with my head wedged under the window handle.

20 May – Up at 4am and we started off an hour later. The Colonel rampaged because it was not earlier. There was a fine drizzle when we set off which soon turned into a heavy downpour. We had only 20 miles to cover but the roads were hilly and twisty with the surfaces pitted with shell holes and all the bridges blown. We crossed the Garigliano river over a pontoon bridge which swayed under the weight of the heavy lorries. Beyond the river we climbed up a steep hill and through what was left of St Georgia, which was nothing but rubble. The last few miles were a nightmare. The deep shell holes had been churned up and turned into craters of mud by the traffic and rain and it was impossible to see them until it was too late. We all fell into them in turn and had to be pulled out by the breakdown truck.

This time we were camped in a flat field deep in grass and flowers. Yantze, our radiologist, was our first casualty. He had flung himself down in the grass for a five minute rest and was run over by one of the water buggies, which never saw him in the long grass. He let out a blood-curdling yell and we thought that he must be dead. Not at all –

amazingly he was only bruised and badly shaken. He had been pancaked into the soft mud and the weight of the buggy and his portly figure had left a deep depression in the ground.

It was much hotter here than at St Georgia. At St Clemente we were in a valley surrounded by hills; to our right we could see Monte Cassino and beyond the Monastery were snow-capped mountains.

The Germans were clearly visible on our left, and behind and all around us the divisional artillery were siting their guns. Two of their heavy guns were only a few yards from the hospital tents. We had been pushed this far forward so that we would not be left behind as quickly as the last time, nor would we have to send out a forward unit. The Colonel told us, as if it were a joke, that if we were shelled we could not claim protection from the Geneva Convention as we were beyond the safety limit laid down for hospitals, and we had to take down our Red Cross signs.

Shelling started up quite soon after we had installed ourselves, and continued for several days. We could clearly see the projectiles whizzing over in each direction. Recce planes attached to the division flew over our heads and the rumble of tanks trundling along the road below our field added to the noise, as did the bombers unloading their bombs a few fields away. The puffs from the ack-ack guns fired at them looked like balls of cotton wool in the sky.

Biddy and I shared a tent and she woke me up the first night, shouting to me to get out because shrapnel was coming in, but it was only fire-flies. We laughed about it afterwards but it showed how bomb-happy we were becoming.

Early next morning the wounded started arriving again and I was back in the resuscitation tent with Margaret. We were shelled for an unpleasant half hour during our lunch break and had a lucky escape. We had all just sat down at our open air mess table when the Colonel called us to come and help unload a newly arrived convoy of ambulances. When we returned for our lunch an hour later the table was a shambles; there was a huge hole in the middle and mugs and plates all over the place with bits of shrapnel sticking out of them. Another shell had landed near our tent but had not exploded. Several of the hospital tents had holes in them and a large piece of shrapnel had flown through one of the operating tents. No one was in it at the time and miraculously not one of the hospital staff was hurt.

Two days later I set off early to collect the NAAFI and post. I had been told that Cassino had fallen to the Allies during the night and decided to go through it on my way to Casserta and save several miles.

Cassino, immediately after its capture, was the saddest sight I ever saw. Never before, or since, have I seen a town razed to the ground so completely. It was worse than Tobruk or Oradour, a French town razed by the Germans to rubble, and every one of its inhabitants killed. Cassino looked like a rabbit warren, with holes in the rubble where soldiers had taken refuge. It was impossible to know where the streets or houses had been. Even the little stream running alongside the bottom of the town had been bombed out of its bed and wandered aimlessly around. The surrounding hills looked as if they had been swept by a hurricane; once covered with trees, they were now blackened by fire. The few still left standing had broken trunks and branches hanging down in grotesque positions which made them look like an army of phantoms.

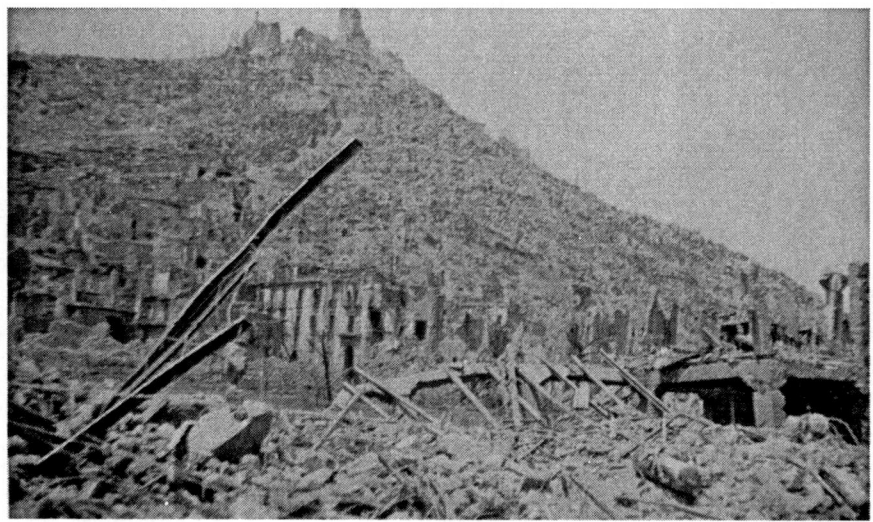

The town and monastery of Monte Cassino the day after it fell to the Allies.

The monastery, perched on top of the hill overlooking the town like a sentinel, had also been bombed and shelled into ruins. From its position one could well imagine what an impregnable fortress it had been for the Germans and how difficult to storm from below.

The shell holes and bomb craters made travelling along the road extremely slow and difficult, especially as there was a steady stream of armour coming towards me on its way to the front. I collected the post from Vallona and the NAAFI from Casserta, where I managed to get a month's supply of whisky and gin. I called in on a friendly Canadian bakery where they gave me 24 pounds of fresh white bread, a pleasant change from our hard black army loaves.

I missed the turning off the road to the pontoon bridge beyond Cassino and continued up the road without realising my mistake. Suddenly a tank blew up in front of me. I had pulled over to the verge to let another tank pass and it ran over a mine. I reversed as quickly as I was able to. The crew threw themselves out of the tank just before it caught fire, and ran down the road. The ammunition started exploding, scattering shells and shrapnel all over the place. Some bits clanged against my car and broke a window.

At this moment a Military Policeman drove up on a motor bike: 'Where the hell do you think you're going? The Germans are just ahead beyond the bend in the road.' I turned round quickly and took the only soldier who had been wounded to a CCS a mile down the road. Two miles further down I found the track leading to the pontoon bridge. It was not surprising that I had missed it as there was no sign. An enormous crater had appeared in the road since I went down it a few hours before.

Immediately after I had wobbled over the bridge and on to the track again a spotter plane crash-landed in front of me, completely blocking my track. The pilot was not hurt and I helped him out of the cockpit and gave him a drink of whisky from my supplies. He helped me drive the car round his plane, which meant going into the ditch and out again. I took him back to the hospital with me from where he was able to radio for help.

Five minutes after I arrived back at the hospital it was shelled again. Just as I was distributing the NAAFI to three of the Quakers, they all dived under a nearby truck without any warning. I was so surprised at their sudden disappearance that I did not realise what was happening and stupidly continued to sit on the edge of my car until someone shouted at me to put on my tin hat and get down. The shells made a nasty whistle as they passed overhead. One from this attack fell near Kelsey, who was taking a nap in the sun outside her tent, and blew her off her chair. Both the mobile theatre and Michael Rowntree's biscuit tin of a van had bits blown out of them. Another shell went straight through the theatre tent where the Colonel was operating on an abdominal. He calmly told the orderlies to move the patient from the operating table to the ground and continued operating. As he spread the intestines on the grass looking for perforations Jean Barr, his theatre sister, just missed stepping on them as she returned with some instrument he needed. I'm glad to say the patient recovered completely and was never told of the danger he had been in. We always wondered how much grass went back into his abdominal cavity together with his guts.

We four drivers had now completed our 15 days' CB and were able to entertain and be entertained again. Tommy came over several times and Biddy got the odd day's leave to be with him. We were not shelled again. The Germans had been pushed back and our guns had moved out after them. A few days later our division was pulled out of the line for a rest and fewer wounded arrived. During the time our division had been in action we received 750 wounded while we were at St

Clemente and 630 at St Georgia, apart from those who were treated by our forward unit and evacuated direct to the base hospitals.

Three of our staff were wounded by the shelling, but none seriously. One of the wounded FAU walked about with two inches of bandage neatly showing above his stocking. He was still wearing it several weeks later when Rome had been liberated; he hopped a lift into Rome whenever he could, drawing attention from the Italians as a wounded soldier, thereby collecting sympathy. I got fed up with his performance and asked the Colonel how bad his injury was. The Colonel said: 'It's just a mosquito bite'. With that information Kit and I scrounged a dilapidated baby's pram and left it outside his tent with a message: 'Next time you go to Rome you must use this'. Miraculously the bandage came off the following day and he was back on duty. He was the only one of the COs who was really objectionable.

28 May – The division moved up to the front line again and took part in the allied attack on Rome. A forward unit was sent up to the division while we closed the hospital. We received a visit from the American general in charge of the Mediterranean Medical Corps. We were ordered to put on our best uniforms and polish our belts and buttons – something we never did gladly. The General had lunch with us and the meal dragged on until mid-afternoon – to everyone's disgust as we had better things to do.

Three days later we received orders that we were not to move until 2 June as the division had been put on virtual 'standby'. We learnt much later that they had been halted in their tracks to allow the Americans the honour of entering Rome at the head of the Allied armies.

As we had nothing much to do, Kit and I took the sisters Kelsey, Margaret and Mary for a trip to the sea. All the sisters had been working without a break since the division had gone into action. None of them had been able to leave the hospital – unlike us, who were always able to find an excuse to get out and away in our cars. We drove through Pontecorvo, which had fallen to the Free French and Canadians who were fighting alongside each other. The town lay on the side of a hill and had been the scene of bitter fighting; it was finally captured on the twenty-sixth. Five days later the German dead had still not been collected for burial and were lying everywhere, grotesquely swollen by the heat and covered in flies, stinking to high heaven. The carcasses of their horses, still harnessed to their carts, lay between the broken tanks and lorries.

We drove on through Pica and climbed a steep hill to the deserted monastery of Monte Lencio. We entered the church, the structure of which was undamaged. Altar cloths and richly embroidered vestments had been torn to pieces and covered with human excrement. Beautiful old illuminated manuscripts had been ripped apart and their pages used as lavatory paper. Dirt and excreta had been smeared on all the Holy pictures and frescoes. Crucifixes and chalices had been smashed and the altar itself hacked down. It was a sickening sight and we wondered which army had been responsible.

We did not feel like any more sightseeing after this and drove over the hill, down the other side and across marshy tracks to the sea. We ate our army ration picnic there, swam in the clear blue sea and felt clean again.

2 June – We set off in convoy – as usual, over a bad road. Some of the convoy got lost and joined a Canadian unit whose army number was the same as ours – 54. We collected a number of Canadian trucks which had made the same mistake. We were held up for quite a time by a British truck loaded with smoke bombs and hand grenades which was on fire. We were not allowed to pass it until it had burnt itself and its ammunition out. We parked ourselves on the side of a hill two miles north of Ceccano. The hospital was not unpacked as we were only in transit, but we were given our own tents and camp beds.

Iris and I left the camp early on the morning of 3 June for Naples. Iris was to collect her car which the REME workshop was repairing for her, and I needed to collect the post, stores, *etc*. We went first to the *Hotel Patria* and booked ourselves in for the night as we had too much to do in one day. We then went to collect 76, and I managed to scrounge a new carburettor and distributor for 82. It was dark by now and we returned to the hotel for a meal and bed.

4 June – Rose at 5am. Iris returned to the hospital and I went to the officers' shop, NAAFI and post. I found a market open and bought strawberries and cherries for the mess. I reached Ceccano by midday and could see the hospital getting into its convoy line ready to move off. I was on the wrong side of the river and found, to my dismay, that the only bridge (which we had crossed the day before) had been blown up an hour before I had reached it and no one knew of another way across. A Canadian MP sent me back to Frossinone, saying I could get over a bridge there, but when I arrived it had just been blown up. I was sent to a series of small roads leading to nowhere by more Canadians until I got fed up and went to the Canadian HQ and asked for a guide. They produced a sergeant with a jeep who said he knew of a ford. By this time I had been joined by two Canadian trucks who had also lost their way trying to get over the river. They had followed me, again mistaking my number for their own.

The sergeant took us across open fields, in ever widening circles, until he had to admit that he could not find the ford. By this time I was desperate as I knew that the hospital must have left and I had no idea where they were going. I left the sergeant and trucks and got back on to a sort of road and drove down it as fast as I could until I came to a posse of soldiers guarding a barricade. They were waving their arms like mad as I approached. When I reached them I asked them what was the matter and they said I had just driven down a road which was mined and that they were waiting for the Sappers to de-mine it. Either I was lucky or there were no mines. I continued on my way and returned to Poji along a one-track lane until I came to a truck stuck in the mud half way up a hill. There was no way round it and I wasted another hour helping them to dig it out. When I finally reached Poji another MP tried to send me back on the wrong road. This time I ignored him and continued in the direction of the river until I came to a perpendicular hill leading to a ford across the river. I went down it in bottom gear with both the hand and foot brake on. When I reached the bottom 82 stood on her head. I did not know whether another rev would turn her over, and slowly released the brakes and gently accelerated. She kindly righted herself and we drove through the ford. The hill on the other side was almost as steep as the one we had come down and I did not think she would be able to climb it in the mud. With the help of a stone behind her back wheels as we started off, and she made it.

I finally reached the hospital site to find it empty except for two Quakers collecting the last bits. They told me the route the convoy had taken and where they were heading for.

I set off in pursuit and hadn't gone many miles when my radiator started to boil over. I discovered that water was leaking from the tap which had probably been damaged when 82 stood on her head. While I was trying to tighten it a burly French Légionnaire came by and offered to help, saying that it needed a strong man to turn it. He gave it a terrific twist and pulled the whole tap off. A flood of boiling water poured out. I thanked him kindly and sent him on his way. I collected a handful of sticks from a nearby hedge and whittled one down to wedge in the hole. Miraculously it stayed there. I filled up the radiator from one of the jerry cans we always carried with us and continued on my way. The traffic became more and more intense; two large convoys of Canadians were muddled up with our division and it was difficult to pass because of the oncoming vehicles. I eventually caught up with the hospital, which was more or less stationary, at sunset. They were moving only three or four yards every quarter of an hour. They were delighted to get their post and to eat the strawberries and cherries. We continued at this dreary pace until we crossed Route 6 – the main Rome-to-Naples road – when our speed increased. It was quite dark by then and difficult to see the road without lights and through all the dust thrown up by the vehicles in front. I had been driving since six o'clock that morning and was exhausted. I must have dozed off as I woke up with a tremendous bump to discover that I had driven off the road before a bridge and was stuck in the sand of a dried-up river bed. I was so tired that I hoped I would be left there and allowed to sleep until the breakdown lorry came along – but no, I was heaved out by one of the water buggies and put on the road again. We eventually halted at midnight at a most palatial building which we were told was the agricultural college of Palestrina. I flopped down on my flea-bag, too tired to drink the hot soup which our devoted cooks always provided at the end of a convoy drive. This was one of my worst driving experiences – until we reached France when the snow posed problems of its own.

9

TO ROME AND THE VATICAN

Next morning I drove 82 to the Atelier Lourd where, within an hour, they soldered my radiator tap back for me and put on two new tyres. Meanwhile, Biddy had collected our bedding and found two rooms away from the others and underneath the eaves in the attics. I was woken early the next morning by the sounds of hens cackling somewhere nearby. Biddy said I was imagining things but I followed the sounds and managed to open a door leading to the attic where, hidden in the rafters, I found about two dozen hens. I collected a dozen eggs for breakfast. I suggested to the Colonel that we had roast chicken for lunch but he said no; they obviously belonged to the caretaker who had hidden them from the pillaging soldiers. This was true and I told the caretaker to collect them and put them somewhere out of earshot. He was so grateful that we had not eaten them all – no thanks to me – that he supplied us with eggs until we moved on.

Three days later I drove Solly Albert, Père Boileau, Aboucher and Frankau to Rome which had been liberated by the Americans as planned. It was only 35 kilometres from Palestrina but it took us a good hour to get there because of all the military traffic and shell holes in the road which had to be avoided. Père Boileau and I visited the Vatican and St Peters, his first visit and mine. We were suitably impressed by the Pope's high altar, the stained glass windows, the effigies of all the previous Popes, and by the size of St Peters. The statue of St Paul in black stone with his foot worn away by the pilgrims' kisses was particularly moving, but what moved me most was Michaelangelo's marble Pietà. We visited the rooms of Raphael in the Vatican and last of all, and the most awe-inspiring, the Sistine Chapel with Michelangelo's ceiling. I was so glad that we were able to see it on our own, wandering where we pleased. We returned to the others and wandered around Rome. We saw the church with the twelve Michelangelo apostles on its roof, the extraordinary monument of Victor Emanuel, the Gardens of the Seven Hills of Rome and the Victory Monument to Garibaldi. We had time to wander through the shopping area; very few shops were open but I was able to buy some films and photographs. About eight kilometres from Palestrina 82 broke down and I had to get a tow back.

11 June – Wherever we parked our cars beggars arrived from nowhere – every bit as ragged and miserable as the poorest Egyptians. We

packed up and got our cars ready, even finding time to decorate them with flowers. We left at midday, by-passing Rome. The roads were lined with Italians waving and cheering and throwing flowers at us. We wondered if they liked us any better than the Germans, and whether they had cheered them more or less enthusiastically.

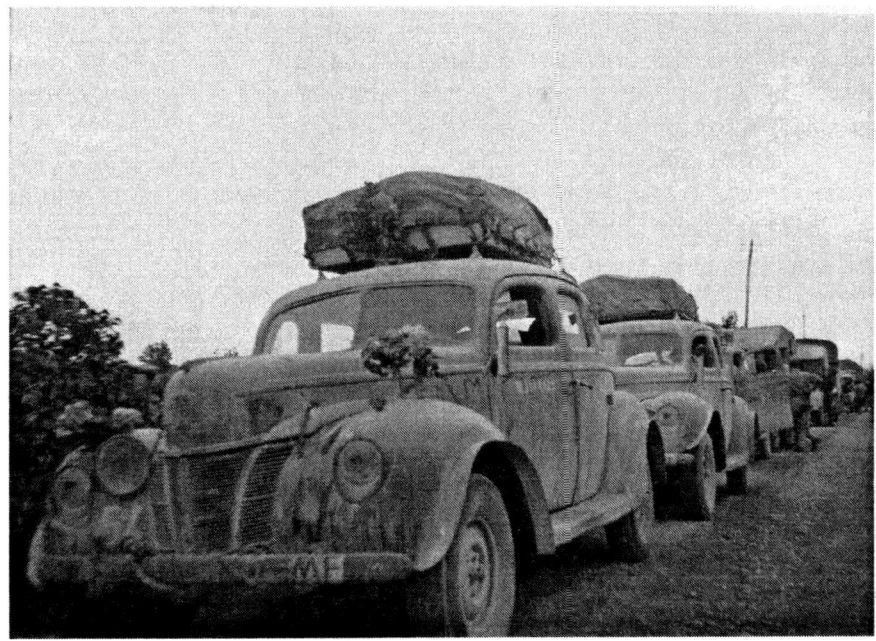

Italy – convoy with flowers.

We left Palestrina in convoy at 1pm. We drove through Zoparol, Tivoli (where we reached Route 6, a much larger road), Baccano, Sutri, Coprani and stopped about three kilometres outside Viterbo. The country was flat and uninteresting until we reached Sutri where we climbed up and around rocky hills with villages perched on top of them; sometimes a castle as well. We drove past a small lake, after which we started to see signs of war and carnage – dead German soldiers and horses, and burnt out tanks and vehicles. We reached a flat piece of ground at 7pm in total darkness.

We slept on the ground alongside our cars. An awful stench near my car kept me awake, but it was too dark to investigate. As soon as it was light I discovered that I had been lying between a dead German and a dead horse. The buzzing of the flies around them and the smell made it impossible for me to stay there a minute longer and I moved my car out of range.

After breakfast I drove the Colonel, Jean Barr and Michael Rowntree to try and find a better site for the hospital – but we failed. There were dead Germans all along the roadside. The Colonel made me stop the car several times to look at them; he seemed to take a delight in watching our reactions. They were a nauseating sight; their putrefying bodies blackened and bloated by the heat, covered with flies and with that sickening sweet smell of death. When the Colonel drew our attention to the maggots crawling out of their ears and nostrils both Jean and I started to retch.

By the time we returned to the field the dead Germans and horses had been removed and buried. The Colonel gave the order for the tents to be put up immediately and the hospital opened to receive the wounded, who had already started to arrive.

During the next four days we received 250 wounded. A bitter battle was fought around Montefiascone which cost our division heavy losses and I was back to the resuscitation ward. The Colonel of the Fusilier Marins, Le Capitaine de Fegate Amyot d'Inville, who was one of de Gaulle's original Free French officers, was blown up in his jeep near a destroyed bridge. At least a dozen vehicles had been down the detour around the bridge before he went over – in fact it was René who reached the bridge first with his squadron of scout cars. He suspected mines and sent word back for the sappers to check and clear a path. Unfortunately d'Inville arrived before they did so, hit a mine, and was blown straight out of his jeep and killed instantly. The mine was a new type, made of plastic and timed to explode after a number of vehicles had driven over it.

The body of his Colonel had barely reached the hospital when René himself was brought in with a piece of shrapnel in his thigh. He was lucky – the shell hit the engine of his jeep where most of it lodged.

Montefiascone was captured and the division continued its attack toward Bolsena and Orvieto. By the fifteenth we had been left well behind again and received orders to evacuate the wounded, pack up and move on. Coupigny was sent in the direction of Bolsena with a forward unit and we sat in our cars waiting for the order to move.

Our movement orders arrived at last and we were told to join Coupigny on the shores of Lake Bolsena. The drive only took two hours but we had to wait for the Italian peasants to finish harvesting their corn – with our help – before we could put up our tents on a nice flat piece of ground alongside this beautiful lake.

The hospital was machine-gunned by enemy planes during the night and, although no one was hit, there were plenty of holes in the tents. The hospital soon filled up with military and civilian casualties. Two more popular and gallant Free French officers were killed during this attack. Captain Meza of the 22nd BNNA and Colonel Champrosy, Commander of the Artillery. Champrosy was dead when he reached the hospital and Meza died soon afterwards. René was wounded and evacuated to a base hospital. Mazières, who took over René's squadron, was wounded in turn and lost an eye; Prazybilaki, who took over from him, was badly burnt on his face and legs when his scout car was hit by a shell and burst into flames.

During this time we also admitted Italian civilian wounded and eventually had to put up a tent of forty beds for them. The very first to arrive was a mother with her two-year old child. The mother had multiple wounds and both the child's arms were shattered. In spite of the blood transfusions I gave them, they both died.

Little by little the division was withdrawn from the front line and the number of wounded decreased. The convoys of ambulances arrived empty and came to evacuate our patients further south to the base hospitals.

18 June – Lady Spears arrived at Naples. Kit drove down to collect her and brought her back to us the following day. We were delighted to see her again and to win her approval. General Juin paid us a visit on 21 June and told us that the Division was to be sent down to the south of Italy for leave and to re-group before being sent to France. This news made the French delirious with joy at the thought of returning to their country, no longer as outlaws but as liberators.

Another day General Brosset turned up with a Comtesse de Luart who was with a mobile hospital attached to the North African division. We envied her smart navy uniform and silk stockings and high-heeled shoes. We never heard of her again or whether she took her ambulance to France.

We spent several weeks at Lake Bolsena and made ourselves quite comfortable. It rained quite a lot, but it was so warm that we dried out quickly, and we had all been issued with gumboots and macs. We did all our washing in the lake and bathed there too. The lake had a sandy shore and bottom and was quite shallow for several yards. The Italians brought their beautiful white, velvet-eyed oxen to water at the lakeside in the evenings and fished from boats in the middle of the lake. Bullfrogs croaked all night in the reeds but we soon got used to their booming. Surprisingly there were no mosquitoes.

We all appreciated this fairly peaceful time with the hospital less than half full of patients and being reduced daily. We needed the rest. From the day that the division went into action on the Garigliano river we had moved camp every four or five days and frequently found a fleet of ambulances waiting for us when we arrived.

During the comparatively short time since we arrived in Italy we were deployed eight times and advanced over 1,000 kilometres. We admitted 2,702 patients, of whom 2,000 were wounded in action. The lists showed that 2,518 were from our own division, 48 were American,

18 British from the Eighth Army, 40 German prisoners and, finally, 78 Italian civilians wounded in cross-fire.

We had four surgical teams who operated non-stop, except when we were in convoy. There were 251 major operations between 11 May and 20 June, including 48 abdominals, 9 open thorax, 21 amputations, 3 tracheotomies and 4 severe burns.

During the campaign 700 operations were completed, all of first or second urgency. In the resuscitation ward we gave 1,500 litres of plasma and 480 blood transfusions. We did not have one case of either tetanus or gas gangrene amongst the military wounded. One Italian woman died of gas gangrene and one baby of tetanus, both of them dying within a few hours of admission.

We had 86 deaths – 77 Frenchmen, 6 Italians, 2 Germans and 1 American. A quarter of these died on admission before we had time to transfuse them or operate. Some were dead on arrival.

This campaign had been particularly severe for the Free French who had little means of replacing their losses; every original Free Frenchman was irreplaceable. In 45 days of combat, the Division lost 700 dead (including 50 officers), and 2,000 wounded (including 200 officers, most of whom had been fighting with the Division since June 1941).

One day, while we were at Bolsena, Kit and I drove Lady Spears to Rome; I took her to shop where I had discovered they sold nylon stockings, make-up and scent. We had lunch at the French Officers' Club and wandered around the Vatican City and ancient Rome.

Two or three days later Ian Calvacoressi, one of General Leese's ADCs, turned up with an invitation for Lady Spears, Kit and me to visit the General at his Eighth Army HQ. It took us two-and-a-half hours to get there over the most awful roads, the surface non-existent in places. We were lucky to have only one puncture. We climbed up narrow, steep, twisty mountain roads to Orvieto where we stopped for a few minutes to admire the superb view over hills and valleys golden with ripe corn. General Leese's HQ was a few miles beyond Ficulla on the side of a hill overlooking a lake and near the ancient town of Perugia. Upon our arrival we were shown to our sleeping quarters – a caravan each with a proper bed, furniture, chintz curtains over the windows, and a wash basin with hot and cold water taps which worked. Drinks were brought to us by an orderly before dinner.

Dinner was in an enormous tent with a bar at one end and comfortable armchairs to sit in. The dining table was laid with white tablecloth and napkins, flowers, silver, cut glass and china; our eyes goggled. The general staff were all assembled – there were dozens of them. We were introduced and knew a few, including David Butters, Sidney Kent and Ian Calvacoressi. It was a dinner of many courses, amusing conversation, several unkind jokes about the Americans, and some odd war stories. General Leese left us as soon as dinner was over, but we remained talking until midnight.

The night was pretty noisy, with shell and gunfire waking up all the nearby cockerels who crowed incessantly. We were called in the morning with early morning tea by a chatty corporal and then breakfasted with General Leese, who then took us for a conducted tour of his own quarters. These consisted of three caravans, bedroom, sitting room and office and map room. He showed us the latest battle movements on the maps. After this we said our farewells and Kit paddled off to see what spares she could wangle from the REME. Lady Spears and I had time to pay a quick visit to the cathedral at Orvieto. The town is enclosed by a high wall dating back to medieval times; we wandered down the old narrow streets, where the houses almost touch each other across the road. They were bright with roses climbing up the walls and geraniums hanging down from window boxes.

We got back to the hospital at midday and found them busy dismantling the tents and packing up. During our absence the order had come through that we were to join the divisional convoy back down to the south of Italy. We were all ready and in line by 7pm but did not actually set off until 9 o'clock, with nothing to guide us but the reflector of the vehicle in front. We had a long wait at Viterbo for the other units to join us, and by-passed Rome arriving at Sandandia near Pittoria at daybreak. Sandandia was one of the new towns built by Mussolini out of the Pontine marshes with much advertisement and fanfare before the war. It had miraculously escaped the violent bombardment and destruction which most of the coastal towns had suffered in that part of Italy. We lodged for the day in the Fascist Naval Academy which had been abandoned by the Italian navy.

We did our best to get some sleep. There were no blinds to stop the strong sunlight from coming through the windows, and the combination of the Benzedrine the Colonel had given us during the previous night's drive, and the sound of vehicles continuously arriving and departing, to say nothing of an endless trail of people barging into our rooms (including a very aggressive American GI who refused to leave until we sent for help from the Colonel), we were prevented from even shutting our eyes. After a few hours we all gave up trying and checked our cars instead.

Our departure from Sandandia was at midnight. We were still part of the divisional convoy and still not allowed any lights, although we were well out of the battle area. We arrived, all in one piece, at 6am at Albanova, where we had spent several weeks on our arrival from Tunisia before the attack on the Garigliano river.

This time we were dispersed in a corn field which was in the process of being harvested. The golden sheaves were piled into stooks under cool lime trees, and vines hung from tree to tree. An almost peaceful serenity penetrated this region of Italy now that the war had moved so far away. We bought baskets of apples and apricots from neighbouring farms, as well as figs, legs of Parma ham, cheese and butter from the markets. We invited our friends to elevenses – beer and slices of army bread spread with butter and ham.

The hospital opened again. This time most of the patients were medical with a high preponderance of VD (Naples Pox); Solly Albert looked after them in a special tent. One of our jobs was to take jars of test tubes to the Pasteur Institute in Naples for Wassermann tests and return with the results. The surgeons still had the odd operation to do, road accidents and wounds caused by brawls with the US army, mostly from their MPs who seemed to be particularly aggressive towards the Free French.

The Colonel took the opportunity to operate on a number of lightly wounded, not serious enough to be hospitalised during the heat of the battle. He removed bits of shrapnel and bullets and tidied up old wounds, mostly for officers who had refused to be parted from their men during an attack.

The day after our arrival I drove Lady Spears, the Colonel and Jean to a review of his troops by General de Gaulle. We got there at 4pm and de Gaulle did not arrive until 6pm. It was very hot indeed and de Gaulle did not even get out of his jeep, but drove at great speed between the lines kicking up clouds of dust. No one was very pleased, least of all Lady Spears of whom he took no notice at all; she took this as a personal insult to her husband. We had an awful drive back trying to pass the slow convoys along dusty roads, every bit as bad as the desert and just as hot. Soon after this the Americans sprayed oil on the untarmacked roads to help to lay the dust.

Another day Lady Spears, the Colonel, Michael Rowntree and I lunched with Admiral Kirk in the palace that King Leopold had built for his mistress near Naples. We lunched in great pomp, with a silk table cloth on the dining-room table and a white-gloved liveried footman behind every chair.

Lady Spears flew back to Beyrouth on 11 July and we did not see her again until we were in Alsace in December.

Our rest period gave us time to look back over the past weeks and digest our experiences. This was the first time we had had German wounded in many numbers in the hospital. The difference in attitudes towards them from the staff swung from one extreme to the other. We thought that several FAU orderlies, who were not Quakers, were actively pro-German. I always presumed that this was why they were conscientious objectors. I disliked having them working for me in my ward and, when I could, had them moved, but this was not always possible.

I had one such orderly, who shall be nameless, when there were five Germans in my ward amongst the 30 odd wounded. One morning I found him washing the feet of all the Germans, saying that he was making them comfortable. This was fair enough, but when I asked him if he was going to do the same for the rest of the patients he replied that it was not necessary as they did not have the same high standard of hygiene. I then discovered that he had given all the spare pillows to the Germans, as well as our only two air cushions and three bed rests. I made him collect them all up and give them to the most needy, only one of whom was a German.

Another time and in a different ward where I had one German patient, I returned after lunch to find the same orderly, who was not working in my ward, talking German to my patient. When he saw me he came across and said that he had come to find out if the German needed anything and would I please see that he had a glass of water by his bed, and he would call in when he was off duty to give the German a blanket bath. This time I really lost my temper. I told him that if he returned to my ward I would report him to the Colonel and have him put on detention. Incidentally, the German had been operated upon the day before for innumerable perforations of the intestines and was not allowed anything by mouth. He was much too ill and shocked to have a blanket bath. He did recover.

To be fair to the Germans they rarely complained and were very courageous. I think that they appreciated the fact that they were treated exactly the same as all the other wounded and given the best possible treatment under difficult conditions. Two rabid Nazis (SS officers) died in my ward when we reached France. They both needed blood transfusions to save their lives but, because I could not – and would not – give my word that the blood was pure Aryan, they both refused them.

We always tried to put the Germans next to each other when we could so that they would feel less isolated. I never saw an act of antagonism displayed to them from any of our own wounded – indeed, a French soldier would share his meagre ration of cigarettes and chocolate with them.

Among the French personnel of the hospital there were two who could not bear to have any contact with Germans. One was Germaine Sablon. One day, when we were very busy, she was giving drinks of water to the many wounded who were lying on stretchers outside the admission wards, with tears running down her cheeks at the sight of so much suffering. I happened to come out of the resuscitation ward to collect my next patient and saw her holding the head of a soldier while she gave him a drink. The soldier tried to thank her in guttural French which made her realise that he was not one of her *pauvres garçons Français* but German. She dropped his head back on the stretcher with the words '*Sale Boche*' before he had time to drink a drop, and moved on to the next one.

14 July – The hospital celebrated the French 'National Day' with a parade and salute of *le Tricolore*, followed by sports and games for the Africans and a large lunch for everyone. The Capitaines gave an evening party with fireworks and their site lit up with fairy lights. They engaged a very good Napolese pianist to entertain us.

I managed to wangle another 48 hours leave to go to Rome with my two friends Washy Hibbert and Humphrey Weld for a private audience with the Pope. We drove there in an open army truck and were covered in dust by the time we arrived. We managed to get rooms at the RAF transit hotel, which only had cold water to the wash basins.

Next morning we rose early and went round the shops searching for presents to send home. We then went to the Sistine Chapel, the rooms of Raphael and to our audience with Pope Pius. He talked to each of us in turn for about ten minutes, after which he held out his hand to kiss St Peter's ring and presented us with a picture of himself and a rosary, which he blessed. I did not tell him that I was not a Catholic and felt rather guilty about accepting the rosary, so I gave it to Weld for his children.

We ended our day by visiting more museums and churches. At the time I did not appreciate how lucky we were in having the unique privilege of visiting all the treasures of Rome without payment, queuing or sharing with other tourists, and being able to enter places which were usually closed to the general public. Our uniforms were sufficient passports to open all doors and we accepted it as our right.

17 July – In the morning, I drove the Colonel to the other side of Montefiascone to find a new site nearer the division. He decided on an uncut cornfield. I got back at 10 and drove Kit to the ACL and later Jocelyn. I then changed the tyres of 82 again. Jean turned up with bruises and a cut lip which needed four stitches; the Colonel had smashed his car (once again) with her in it. I saw the wreck the next day, it was completely written off and a miracle that neither of them had been killed. The Colonel escaped without a scratch. Coupigny and Thibaux left in the evening to guard our site.

19 July – Iris helped me to change the radiator on 82. I listened on my wireless to Ocean Swell winning the Derby. I drove the Colonel to QJ50 and my newly-fitted radiator blew up and I had to get a tow to

the ACL. A sergeant drove me back to the hospital as I had to leave 82 there for the night.

As we were told that we were not staying at Bolsena for more than a few days only two hospital ward tents were put up and we slept outside on our camp beds. It rained and we, and our bedding, got soaked.

The division was still fighting hard, mopping up pockets of Germans on the hills surrounding Montefiascone before attacking Radiocafone and Casciano di Bagni at the entrance of Tuscany. The Foreign Legion and the 22ième Bataillon de Marche, with the support of the artillery, bore the brunt of the operation.

We were all given forty-eight hours' leave. Biddy, Kit and I were given our two days together and decided to drive down to the south of Italy to see if we could get over to the Island of Capri which was out of bounds to the Allied armies. We set off in my car in the early morning of the twelfth. Our first stop was Pompeii, where we wandered around the empty ruins, marvelling at the mosaics and frescoes and the architecture of the houses and streets. We collected bits of lava and mosaic on our way and listened to the history from the guide who attached himself to us and tried to sell us pornographic pictures of brothel frescoes.

The road followed the sea for most of the way. It was very narrow and twisty and it was lucky for us that there was very little traffic – no private cars, just the odd lorry or bullock cart. We passed vineyards with the vines prettily draped over poles, large vegetable gardens and orchards. We passed through small villages which looked very poor, as did their inhabitants. There were very few young men or women. The women were dressed in black with shawls over their heads, looking weary and apprehensive.

Just before Sorrento I took a turning to the right leading to the sea. It was a very narrow twisty lane and halfway down my brakes failed and our speed increased. Kit, who had been dozing in the back, woke up and said: 'What's the hurry?' I replied: 'There isn't any, but my brakes have gone'. 'Put her into third,' said Kit. 'I've done that,' I said. 'Turn off the engine,' said Biddy. 'I've done that too,' I said as our speed increased. As we turned the last corner with the quayside on our right and no barrier between it and the sea, I saw a large rock on my nearside and was able to scrape 82 alongside it and stop. The wing and mudguard were a bit dented and the paint scratched but that was all. It could have been much worse. We found a fisherman willing to row us over the sea to Capri and arranged to meet him the following morning.

I crept back to Sorrento in bottom gear. There was no REME workshop there but Kit managed to mend the brakes and we found some brake fluid in an Italian garage to replace what I'd lost.

A few miles from Sorrento we found a marvellous little restaurant, the Buena Vista, where we had a delicious lunch of langouste, brought out of the sea alive for us to make our choice, rum omelette, fruit and coffee. We continued our sightseeing, winding our way along narrow roads with wooded slopes above us and the deep blue Mediterranean sea below. We were nearly written off twice by ten-ton lorries, the second one missing us by a whisker; in doing so, it crashed into a rock and nearly fell into the sea.

We arrived at Ravello at dusk and found a small empty hotel on the side of a hill, overlooking the sea on three sides. Hot baths and drinks in our rooms before an excellent dinner gave us the impression that we were back to civilisation again.

Breakfast in bed the next morning and, with a picnic lunch provided for us by the hotel, we returned to the harbour where our fisherman was waiting for us with three stalwart friends ready to row us over to Capri. The fishermen sang to us as they rowed. Unfortunately the sea was very choppy and the voyage took much longer than it looked from the shore. Both Kit and I felt seasick. Outside Capri we transferred to a tiny cockleshell which took us between and beneath rocks to the famous Blue Grotto of Capri. We swam in a large subterranean pool of silvery blue water and inspected the stalagmites and stalactites. When we left the Grotto, we returned to our original boat which took us to a long empty sandy beach encircled by empty bathing huts, where we disembarked. We ate our picnic and sunbathed before walking up a series of small paths, winding their way past vine-garlanded villas and gardens gay with bougainvilleas and geraniums.

We reached a small square where we hired a taxi to take us on a tour of the island. We stopped at Dr Axel Munthe's house which, since his death, had been turned into a museum. We were shown round by the caretaker who had been his housekeeper. She told us the history of the house and Dr Munthe's life story. We were also shown the villa of Gracie Fields and peered over the wall to admire her swimming pool before returning to the square where we paid off the taxi. We made our way back down the same little lanes to the beach and our boat. The return journey was much faster, with a calm sea and following wind and tide, with more songs from the sailors. The dinner at Buena Vista consisted of prawns, fish, steak and rum omelette, washed down with Lacryma Christi to complete our very enjoyable holiday.

10

THE GREAT ADVENTURE

3 August – I drove the Colonel to a secret rendezvous with the French Commandos. Being allocated as his driver for that day led to a unique experience in my life. During a picnic lunch among the ruins of Paestum the Colonel was so mysterious about his visit that I was determined to find out what he was up to. The rendezvous was a small fishing village somewhere beyond Salerno. I was left in the mess in charge of a rather amorous Commando messing officer while the Colonel disappeared with the rest of the Commandos in a collection of jeeps. By some delicate questioning, and by pretending that I knew what was going on, I discovered everything I wanted to know about the Colonel's visit and disappearance. On the way back to the hospital I told him what I had found out. He was very taken aback and swore me to secrecy before telling me the whole story.

The Commandos had had severe and often unnecessary casualties when they had landed and captured Elba, largely because they had no medical assistance or equipment with them. They were due to land in the South of France as the spearhead of the invasion, code-named Anvil, and had asked the Colonel to provide a small medical team to accompany them during their disembarkation and remain with them until our division, with our hospital, arrived in France.

The Colonel, with typical enthusiasm, accepted and decided to head the team himself. He had to choose six others to complete his team and was busy going over everyone's qualifications and suitability. I told him how lucky he was and how much I envied him – which was as much polite conversation as anything as it never entered my head that women would be included. The Colonel was silent for a long time and then, to my amazement and slight consternation, said that he didn't see why he couldn't take me as one of his team if he could persuade one of the sisters to come as well. In the meantime I was not to say a word to anyone – it was too secret.

A few days later I spent a weekend in Naples with Humphrey and Washy. During the night I developed an excruciating attack of gyppy tummy; I was in such pain that I thought I must have a burst appendix. An Italian doctor examined me next morning and said it was nothing worse than an attack of dysentery. He gave me an injection which didn't do much good; I managed to drag myself down to the beach at Castelamari but felt so awful that I crawled back to my bed again in the *Hotel Patria*. Next morning we left at dawn. As soon as we reached the hospital I collapsed on to my camp bed. The Colonel dosed me with large amount of sulphanilamide and told me that I had better hurry up and recover as we might be off with the Commandos at any minute. He told me that he had chosen his team of seven. Jean Pryke, for whom he had a soft spot, was his second female. He had wanted our very efficient theatre sister Franka, but she was a Polish Jewess who had escaped from Warsaw where her entire family had disappeared into concentration camps. She very understandably refused because of the possibility of being taken prisoner.

The remainder of our team consisted of Captain Jibery, our head physician who was to be the anaesthetist, Sous-Lieutenant Mergier, our pharmacien, Adjutant Chef Nocceto from the hospital ordnance who was to be in charge of all supplies – medical and rations – and to keep records of all the wounded *etc*, and lastly David Rowlands, one of the Quakers, who would be in charge of sterilisation and surgical instruments, and would assist the Colonel when he was operating. We were all sworn to secrecy and I had to forego the pleasure of telling our friends from various units of the division, when they came to say 'Goodbye' before their departure for France, that we would be there before them.

During our last ten days in Italy Joan and I weathered several storms and alarms before we could be certain that we really were joining the Commandos. The first hurdle was Colonel Bouvet of the Commandos, a charming and battle-scarred Free Frenchman who was later killed in Alsace. He was affectionately nicknamed *Casse Noisette* (nutcracker) because of his jutting chin and decisive manner. He was horrified at the thought of two women joining his élite band. The Colonel and I drove over to see him in his hide-out and succeeded in convincing him that someone had to look after his men after they had been operated upon by the Colonel – and who better than two trained English nurses? After some argument he accepted us and even gave us Commando flashes to put on our sleeves.

Our greatest stumbling block was the Chief Medical Officer of the division, General Geurriac, who had unwillingly given his permission for the Colonel to leave his hospital to aid the Commandos. He adamantly refused to allow the Colonel to include us in his team and told him that there was absolutely no question of any woman being allowed to join the Commandos.

Eventually the Colonel got me to drive him over to the HQ and we bearded the General together. For a good hour he shouted and harangued us. He said that 80% casualties were expected and that if either Jean or I were wounded we would be more trouble than we were worth and that if we were either killed or taken prisoner he would be held responsible, and then he might be involved in an international incident or at least court martialled.

I must admit that I began to get cold feet when he said this, as I had a terror of being taken prisoner. However, I had to say my piece which the Colonel and I had been rehearsing all the way there. I told him that every day women and children were being killed in England by German bombs. That Joan and I had offered our services to the Free French in any way the officer in charge of us thought fit. That as far as my parents and Joan's were concerned he need have no fear; they would never make any trouble. That Joan and I had both volunteered for this particular job – we were both qualified nurses and as I was a driver as well, I could fulfil two roles. Who would nurse the wounded if we were not included? There were no men in our hospital with our qualifications. I concluded by saying that we were both young and tough with no dependants, we were old enough to make our own decisions and would accept full responsibility for ourselves and sign any paper saying so.

The General gave way after this tirade, saying in an injured voice that he did not understand English women; that if we went he knew nothing about it. So that was that. I did not like the idea of 80% casualties one little bit, and had very mixed feelings about winning the argument but it was far too late to draw back now.

Secretly, Joan and I set about getting our things together. We were allowed to take only what we could pack in a small backpack. I waited until Biddy was away driving somewhere to see how much I could stuff into mine. I packed a drill skirt, aertex shirt, change of underclothes, bathing dress, pair of light canvas shoes, and a pair of socks. I also managed to pack a piece of soap, sponge, toothbrush and brush and comb. I decided to travel in drill trousers, bush shirt and desert boots, hang my camera round my neck with my tin hat, and tie a greatcoat round my waist. Last of all I would take my Sam Browne belt with my loaded Biretta revolver and knife attached to it.

Unknown to the Colonel I threw away my Red Cross brassard. The Red Cross convention forbade Red Cross personnel to carry arms, and I had no intention of being taken prisoner. We did not dare pack, so I put all my bits and pieces in my tin trunk.

I was still suffering from dysentery and had become very thin, in spite of all the medicine I was swallowing. I had to rush to the WC every time I drank or ate anything, but the abdominal cramps had gone and I had felt stronger in the last three days.

8 August – I was woken at midnight by an anxious voice asking me if I felt all right and I knew the moment of our departure had arrived. 'We leave at 5am!' the voice said, 'and you will be called by Jean at 4am.' Jean Barr, as head sister, had been let into the secret as she was responsible for Joan and the running of the wards.

Luckily for me Biddy had left that morning on 48-hour leave with her husband Tommy. I tottered round the tent and, with the help of a torch, stuffed the things out of my tin trunk into my backpack. I put out the clothes that I would be wearing, together with my coat, tin hat, camera and belt, on Biddy's bed. I scribbled a note to Biddy saying that by the time she read it I would be beyond recall. She told me later that she was furious at the way I had skipped off without telling her as she was head driver and in charge of us, and should have been told – but that was not my business.

At 4.30am we assembled in the mess with hot, sweet, sticky coffee and biscuits. I felt better but not completely recovered. When we had eaten we loaded ourselves into two jeeps; our four panniers of medical equipment were already loaded on a 15cwt truck.

Our destination was a small fishing village named Agropolis, where I had previously driven the Colonel. While the Commandos continued their training with our officers Joan and I had nothing to do. We were shown our sleeping quarters, in an empty room in an empty school, a row of straw palliasses laid out on the stone floor. No blankets or pillows, but we had our coats if it was cold in the night. We lunched with the Commando officers in their mess; then the Colonel did his exercise with the Commandos and, to finish the day, took us for a ride in his jeep. Round the back of the village and up into the hills we arrived at a small village overlooking the sea, from where we could see three ships lying at anchor, one of which, the Colonel said, was the ship that would take us to France. He was as excited as a small boy. I had never seen him in such good form, or so enthusiastic – he could not stay still for a moment.

Next morning Joan and I lay in bed and the others went down to the sea for a swim. Commandant Montgraham, who looked like a brigand out of a story book, took us to lunch at the Officers' Club in Salerno, introduced us to all the Commando officers, and then took us for a trip to Amalfi.

We were up at 7am the next day, all packed and ready. We waited on the veranda and watched the three ships steam nearer to the shore. They stopped within half a mile and launched a fleet of small craft to collect us.

The Colonel chose this moment to tell Joan and me that the Captain had no idea that there would be any women boarding his ship. We were to do our best to conceal the fact until the ship had got under way – Bizerta all over again, but this time with no make-up. There really wasn't much we could do except push our hair up under our tin hats – mine was very short anyway. We put on our backpacks and helped load the panniers into the boat. We said 'goodbye' to Jean and then clambered into the boat, keeping our mouths shut. Half way to the ship something went wrong with the motor of our boat and we had to transfer to another which took us alongside the *Prince David*, a Canadian liner transformed into a troop carrier, for our transport to France.

Our boat was hauled up the ship's side by pulleys – an alarming experience as it tipped in all directions before arriving level at a deck. There were several cat-calls as we travelled up the side of the ship, but once in the wardroom with the rest of our group, the ship's officers were too busy to take much notice of us. As the Colonel had planned, the Captain didn't learn we were on his ship until we were under way, by which time it was too late for him to do anything.

Our four panniers of medical equipment were carefully stowed away. They had been meticulously packed by the Colonel and reduced to the absolute minimum of 500 kilos. They contained 800 plaster bandages, surgical instruments, ether, bandages, elastoplast, dressings, medicaments, 50 blankets, one steriliser and 20 stretchers. Except for the steriliser the equipment was divided between the four panniers, so that if one was lost it would not be a disaster.

Once the ship's Captain had recovered from the shock of having two females aboard he was extremely kind to us and, I think, rather intrigued by the whole idea. He turned two unfortunate officers out of their comfortable cabin and gave it to us – it was a palace after the straw palliasses and stone floor of the empty school. There were two comfortable bunks, a wash basin, chairs and a library of books. The only complaint we had was that it was unbearably hot, as it was immediately above the engine room and the porthole had been battened down. We had to make do with a small vent and a fan. The food was first class. As soon as we arrived on board we were given hot buttered toast and coffee; lunch was a four-course meal.

The Admiral in charge of the landing operations was on board the *Prince David* and he and the Captain took Jean and me on a conducted tour of the ship, and then to the bridge, and told us that we were welcome there whenever we pleased. We took part in the roll-call with the Commandos after tea, and a press photographer took photographs. The rest of the day we spent in the wardroom or on the bridge.

Next morning after breakfast, and at the reasonable hour of eight o'clock, we went up to the bridge again and watched the ship's progress through the Straits of Medina: Sardinia on our left, Corsica on our right. Soon afterwards we were told that we and the Commandos were to land on Corsica and remain there for 48 hours to enable them to carry out their final assault exercises.

We were the last to leave the ship and so were able to watch the Commandos launch their landing craft, scramble up the beach and disappear. Then it was our turn to be swung over the side of the ship in our craft, lowered to the sea and deposited on the beach – in the Gulf of Valenco, near the small town and port of Porpriano, and completely deserted. This wild and empty corner of Corsica was especially chosen so that the Commandos should have no contact with the inhabitants who, for security reasons, had all been evacuated to another part of the island, except for the odd farmer and shepherd who had animals to tend.

The seven of us left the beach as soon as we had collected ourselves and followed a narrow track which led to a small hollow shaded by olive trees and carpeted with rough grass. Here we decided to set up our camp. The Commandos had given us two guards and we left them in charge while we changed into our bathing dresses and spent the day swimming and sun bathing, only returning to our base in the evening to eat our army rations. We built a fire and boiled some water for coffee in someone's tin hat. A shepherd passed by with his flock of sheep and an irate farmer descended on us claiming that the soldiers had damaged his vines. The Colonel calmed him down, saying that we would not be there much longer and gave him some wine from his water bottle. He then arranged with the farmer that Joan and I would spend the night at his farm as, I think, he was worried that we might be molested by the Commandos. Apart from their officers, they were a pretty rough lot and I don't think he trusted our guards. The Colonel and one of the guards accompanied us to the farmer's house, which was about half a mile away down a track. The farmer's wife was a wrinkled old body who showed no surprise at our arrival. The house was spotlessly clean and Joan and I were given a huge double bed to share in an empty room. Next morning, at daybreak, the farmer escorted us back to the camp. We found everyone in good heart and after breakfast, leaving our guards in charge, we all went for a walk. We followed sheep tracks which wound through boulders and twisted and gnarled oak and olive trees and all sorts of aromatic shrubs, including rosemary and thyme, with wild vines climbing through stunted trees. The sun came up; blue sky, blue sea and the pungent odour of the maquis left an indelible memory. Out to sea our three ships were being added to every hour and by the second evening there was a veritable armada anchored beyond the bay. At dawn on 11 August we re-embarked on to the *Prince David* and, while the Commandos checked their equipment for the last time and the ship sailed with her crew busy at their tasks, I sat in a comfortable chair on deck and watched and counted the extraordinary panorama of ships from tiny MTBs to the largest class of capital ship stretched out around us. Every few minutes the silence would be broken by each ship firing its guns, great spouts of water rising out of the sea as the shells dropped into it. The *Prince David* had her turn and the whole ship shook from the concussion of her guns, the booms followed by the rat-tat of Bofors and machine gun fire. After this exercise all was quiet as the procession of ships sailed slowly towards their destination.

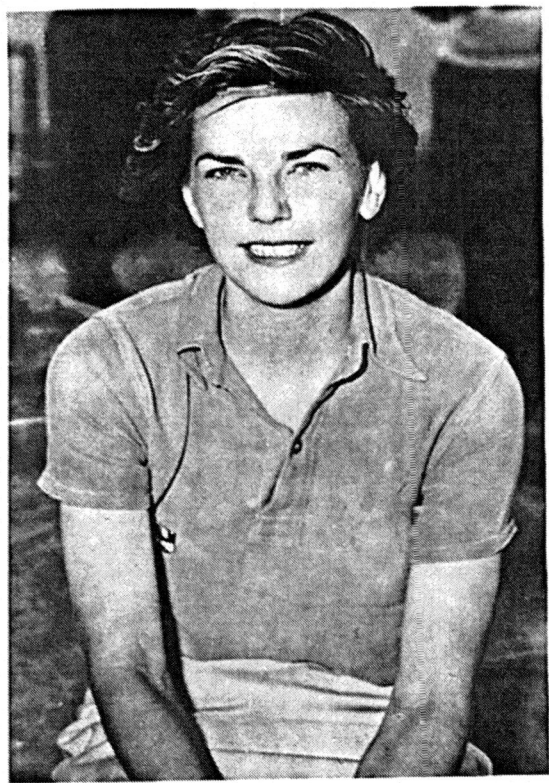

The author on the Prince David *before the Commando landing.*

I spent most of that day alone, reading and wondering what the night held in store for us and thinking how lucky I was to be on this adventure. The Captain invited me to his cabin for tea with his officers and gave me a bottle of Canadian whisky to fortify us. I just managed to stuff it into my haversack, wrapped around with socks and underclothes, and I prayed that I would not fall over and break it. Sunset, and the fleet began to split up, groups stealing away and disappearing over the horizon. By the time darkness fell we, and our two companion ships with their escort of destroyers and MTBs, were alone once more.

Quite soon after darkness had fallen 'action stations' sounded and Joan and I returned to our cabin, packed our belongings and changed into our landing apparel. I threaded my Sam Browne belt through the holster of my Biretta revolver and my knife and then through the dees of my trousers and went up to the wardroom to see what everyone else was doing. I found the ship's doctor busy turning the wardroom into a first-aid centre and helped him lay out his instruments and dressings. He explained to me that during action stations every non-combatant crew member had a special job to do: as medical orderlies, firefighters, feeding shells to the guns and so on. The ship's wireless had been turned off and the entire ship blacked out, with only a few dim blue lights burning inside.

When the doctor had completed his first-aid surgery I returned to my cabin and took off my revolver, which was continually getting in my way, knocking against my hip and pulling my trousers to one side at an uncomfortable angle. I tried to rest but the heat was oppressive and I was too excited so I gave up and, collecting all my things together, climbed up to the wardroom again where I found the rest of our group waiting for supper of soup and sandwiches.

At 9pm the Colonel of the Commandos addressed his men through the ship's Tannoy. In the complete silence and darkness it sounded extremely impressive: '*Attention, attention, les Commandos Français se rassemblent dans une demi-heure sur le pont de leurs embarcations, terminé, terminé.*' The ship's engines had been silent for some time and perhaps because of the total silence everyone spoke in whispers. We went on deck and watched the first wave of Commandos arrange themselves in their boats which were then lowered. The sea was as calm as a pond – no sound except for the creaking of the pulley ropes as the boats were gently launched. We strained our eyes until the little boats were swallowed up in the darkness of the night and listened to the chug of the engines until they were out of earshot.

The first group of Commandos had all been hand-picked and each man had a specific job of work, some to go at all speed to contact the Resistance, others to remain on the beaches and clear a way through the minefields, marking it with white tape. Montgraham, whose house was at Hyères, knew every inch of the territory; with two others he climbed the barefaced rock of Cap Nègre and put out of action the big naval gun sited there facing out to sea.

We had a tense hour to wait until our turn to leave came and I discovered, to my consternation, that my tin hat had disappeared. It had obviously been grabbed by someone who had mislaid his and had already left. Fear born of superstition gripped me and I was certain that this was an omen predicting that I would be popped off – or worse, taken prisoner. The quartermaster kindly replaced my hat with a brand new one but I was not reassured. I had had my old tin hat since I joined the unit and although I was not sentimentally attached to it I did not like losing it at this particular moment.

At 11pm we gathered in the wardroom to be counted and checked and to be given final instructions, after which we groped our way through the darkness and through the many black-out curtains to the boat deck. The seven of us were a curious group, all carrying an amazing collection of bundles slung from our shoulders and all sorts of bits and pieces hanging round our waists. Jibery had slung around his neck a strange oblong-shaped parcel wrapped in a blanket which was to cause him trouble later on when it kept getting caught up in brambles and thorn trees. One of our boat companions was a war correspondent to, I think, *The Times*. He was not at all amused when I told him that he looked like Tweedledee in *Alice Through the Looking Glass*. He had everything except the kitchen stove slung around his fairly corpulent person – a typewriter, saucepan, primus stove, water bottle, binoculars and goodness knows what else. He had some difficulty heaving himself into the boat. Already loaded into the boat was a jeep, our four panniers of medical stores, and the 20 stretchers. Between 30 and 40 people, including us, climbed silently into the boat. Those lucky enough found a seat or perched on the side of the boat; others had to stand. Gently and noiselessly we were lowered into the sea and the engines started. We drifted around for a few minutes waiting for the arrival of three more LCMs and the torpedo boat, which was our escort and pilot.

At last we were all assembled and we moved off to our unknown destination. A pitch black, windless night, a waveless sea, and silence broken only by the pop-pop of the engines and the lapping of the water against the sides of the boat. Smoking and talking were forbidden and no one moved or made a sound as we strained our eyes and ears to see a flare or hear a gun. Slowly we made our way, leaving a trail of phosphorescent water in our wake. The minutes ticked away until faintly, to the left of us, came the muffled sound of guns and the dim light of a flare.

I looked at my watch; almost an hour and a half had passed since we started our journey. Gradually the gunfire became more distinct and we could distinguish the difference between flare and Very light, and then, dimly, the outline of the coast of France appeared out of the blackness.

A quivering and tensing of muscles crept round the boat. When the contours of the coast became clearer our boat pulled away from the other two and sailed right-handed for a short distance before stopping with engines silent. An empty LCM drifted past us but we did not dare call out to it for news. We waited silently a mile off shore for a long half hour, by which time we were all suffering from cramp. I longed for a cigarette. The sky was still cloudless, starless and very black. At last the engines were restarted and, with the engines just ticking over, we slowly made our way to a small cove which we learnt afterwards was Le Canadel, between Le Lavandu and St Raphael. The beach was completely deserted; no lights and no sound of fighting. The moment the boat touched the sandy bottom we scrambled into the shallow water, the drawbridge was lowered for the jeep, which immediately drove away with all our companions including Tweedledee, and the seven of us were left alone.

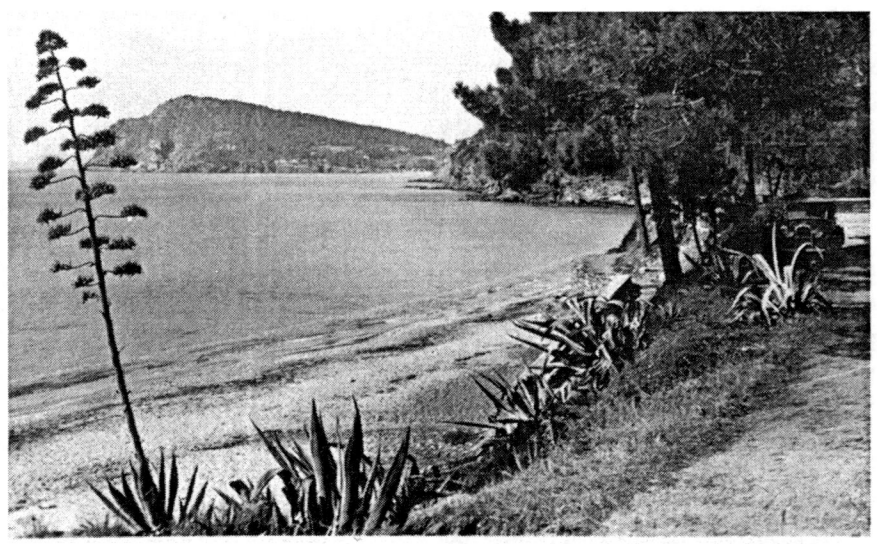

Le Canadel – the 'Commando beach' – where the first wave landed by mistake – luckily. In the background is Le Cap Nègre.

11

ARRIVAL IN FRANCE

For the French to be on French soil again moved them to tears. They all picked up some sand and threw it over their heads. We pulled the panniers and stretchers up the beach and stacked them under a low wall. We left David Rowlands and Nocetto to guard them while the rest of us went in search of the tunnel we had been told was about 500 metres up the railway track. We spent the night there, having collected David and Nocetto, and set up our first-aid unit. We found, without difficulty, the steps leading from the beach to a small path which led us in turn on to the railway line. We cut the wire to get on to the track and turning left, as we had been told to do, walked towards the tunnel. But there was no tunnel and, after covering the 500 metres at least twice, we came to a small railway official's house on the side of the track, with a light burning in one of the windows. After a hurried consultation we decided to risk betrayal and check with the inhabitants the whereabouts of our tunnel. The Colonel took my revolver and cocked it before knocking on the door and we all stood behind him waiting to see what reception we would get and whether they would help or betray us. After several minutes the door opened a crack and a tremulous voice asked in French who was there, while a dog started barking noisily. The Colonel explained in a low voice that we were French Commandos come to liberate them and that we were searching for a tunnel on the railway line.

The door opened wider and, after inspecting us with a spluttering candle, an old man invited us in. I thankfully dropped my backpack, which was beginning to cut into my shoulder, on to the old man's kitchen floor while the Colonel put his question again about the tunnel. The old man shouted for his wife who appeared with a young girl with a baby in her arms which immediately started crying at the sight of us.

The old couple broke down when they heard our story and would not believe that we had arrived by boat a few minutes before. With typical French hospitality they brought us a bottle of white wine and some grapes to eat and we all drank to the liberation of France and to the victory of the Allies. The old man told us that he was a retired railway official who had been allowed to remain in his house in exchange for looking after that section of the line. As far as the tunnel was concerned, it was at least eight kilometres down the line and there was a strong force of Germans guarding the coast between the tunnel and us. We decided that we must have been put on the wrong beach and the Colonel told us to wait in the house while he returned to the boat to find out what had happened.

Hardly had the Colonel departed before he returned with an armed sailor from the boat to say that we had indeed been landed on the wrong beach and that we were to return to the boat with all speed to be re-embarked. The Colonel then disappeared again. Grumbling somewhat, we hoisted our packs on our backs again and trundled off down the railway track after him. Mortar fire and various other sounds of warfare had now begun, and it was getting very noisy. We were half way down the line when the Colonel reappeared to say that the shelling and mortar fire had become too close and accurate for the boat to wait for us to re-embark and, rather than risk it being sunk, which would have done no one any good, the officer in charge had decided to push off. Our instructions were to get away from the beach and coast before dawn as the US Air Force was going to bomb it and to try to reach the Commandos by a roundabout route over the hills, leaving David Rowlands and Nocetto to guard the panniers which we could not take with us.

We returned to the railway house to ask the old man to tell us the quickest way to the hills, avoiding the houses if possible. He told us that it was not difficult to find and hobbled down the track with us to show us a small path which he said would lead to a road which we must follow for half a mile, when we would find a left-handed track leading from it which would take us into the hills.

We started off one behind the other, a pathetic little band, as if we were playing grandmother's footsteps, cursing under our breath if anyone stepped on a noisy twig or kicked a stone. The Colonel led with my revolver in his hand already cocked. The night was still pitch black except when the sky was lit up by flares or Very lights, when we felt naked and instinctively ducked down. When we had covered about a quarter of a mile, we suddenly came upon the road with a horse and cart drawn up on the opposite side. There was no sign of the driver, which made it look even more sinister. The Colonel halted us and crept all the way round it and peered inside. There was no sign of life – very odd, all on its own in the early hours before dawn. Almost immediately after we had crept past the horse and cart we found the path leading up to the hills.

We had not gone many steps along it when the Colonel halted us again and this time we heard guttural voices coming from the other side of a fence bordering the lane. Now we were even more panicky and crawled along the edge of the fence on our hands and knees making, what seemed to me, a painful amount of noise. Luckily there was no dog to bark at us and we got by without being discovered and, huffing and puffing, put a good distance between us and the German camp before we dared get on our feet again.

The path became narrower and narrower until it finally petered out at the bottom of a steep incline. To us, in complete darkness, hampered by our backpacks and bundles which became heavier at every step we took, the climb looked formidable. Trees loomed from nowhere; mimosa, acacia and thorn bushes tore and scratched us and refused to let go of us. Fallen tree trunks tripped us up, rocks grazed and barked our legs, holes swallowed us up without warning. We staggered along like drunks, lurching, falling, slipping, stumbling and halting every few yards to get our breaths. We knew we had until dawn to get out of range of the American bombers.

At one of our halts we heard the sound of approaching footsteps, and each in turn tried to give the correct Commando whistle which we had spent many hours practising. Unfortunately, we were so blown and our mouths so dry, either from thirst or fear, that all we could manage were a few squeaks. In desperation the Colonel called out 'Français' but there was no reply and the footsteps continued to advance. We flattened ourselves to the ground and the Colonel pointed my revolver in the direction the footsteps were coming from but they suddenly veered away and eventually disappeared out of hearing. Had he, whoever it was, seen us? We could see nothing but waited for some time in case the footsteps returned and then continued our climb. Jibery was carrying, as well as his backpack, his curious sausage-shaped bundle which caused him real trouble, as he was perpetually having to disentangle it from the trees.

For our next adventure we almost fell into a cave. The Colonel shone his torch inside which lit up a body. We thought it might be our first patient, but not at all: it was a Commando who had got separated from the main body and, being a sensible fellow, was taking forty winks. He tagged along behind us but could give us no information and had no idea where his unit was. All this time there was a fair bit of gunfire, none if it very near, but every now and then the sky would be lit up and we would crouch to the ground. Fires were raging in the distant hills and the cries of the wounded inter-mingled with shouts, but all too far away for us to reach them and we could not tell whether they were French or German.

By daybreak we had reached the top of the hill and reckoned that we must be well out of range of the US bombers. The Colonel sent Mergier off to reconnoitre and to try to contact the Commandos while we settled down for a rest. We had hardly got ourselves comfortably settled when we heard the sound of aircraft. We sat up and watched as they flew up and down the coastline and then, to our amazement and horror, they turned inland and seemed to make straight for us. 'Lie down,' shouted the Colonel, 'they must have seen us and mistaken us for Germans,' and so it appeared. Each plane, a screaming silver fury, hurtled down towards us, spitting fire from its machine guns and dropping two fish-shaped bombs at the end of its dive. We watched, fascinated, as the bombs spun lower and lower. Just before they landed we put our hands over our ears and waited for the explosion which, when it came, seemed to rock the earth beneath us. Each time there was a lull the Colonel checked our numbers and there was an argument about where the best place was to put one's tin hat – the Frenchmen put theirs over their bottoms! Our Commando friend would change his bush after each attack, like 'Old Bill' in the First World War cartoons: 'If you can find a better 'ole, go to it'. One by one the planes hooked off for good and we emerged from our bushes a good deal dirtier and covered in débris of twigs, stones and clods of earth. The Colonel removed a bit of shrapnel which was embedded in his battle dress top and I had a long cut down my right calf. It was only skin deep and healed up in a couple of days, not even leaving a scar, which was rather disappointing as I would have liked to have been able to show an honourable souvenir of our ordeal. In fact we had a very lucky escape as no one was seriously hurt.

We shared a bottle of water, laced with some of the whisky I had been given, and a packet of American cigarettes, which was all we could find. The Colonel decided that it was time for us to move on again. We had not gone very far when we met two Commando scouts sent from HQ to look for us. They had been afraid that we had either been blown up or taken prisoner and were overjoyed to find us. They told us that HQ was over the next hill and guided us to it, down the farther side of our hill and up another. Now that we could see where we were going walking was much easier; even so it was very much like pushing our way through virgin country. We had to climb over more boulders of rock and wriggle through cascades of brambles and prickly bushes, our backpacks becoming heavier and heavier as their straps cut into our shoulders.

After what seemed to be a very long walk we arrived, panting, at the top of a very steep hill and found HQ installed half way down. While we munched some army biscuits and watched a dog fight overhead, Colonel Bouvet told us that the landing had been 100% successful, a large number of prisoners had been captured, and the Commando casualties were small. They thought there was a suitable house for us to set up our first-aid unit about two kilometres away.

So, once more, we set off, this time downhill. It seemed a very long way. While we were pushing our way through the undergrowth the RAF flew over and dropped a parachute of supplies which landed among the trees – blue, white and yellow, looking like a ballet of balloons. We wanted to stop and collect some but the Colonel said 'No'; we had wasted enough time already and must push on, find our wounded and set up shop. At last we found ourselves alongside a dried-up river bed where the brambles were not so thick, but we still had to zig-zag around rocks and clamber over fallen trees. Jibery got completely tied up in a bramble bush with his bundle and had to be pulled out of it.

By midday we stumbled on to a road, by which time it had become very hot indeed. We sat down by the roadside for a few minutes' rest and it was here that the Colonel remembered the rations he had hidden away and we finished them up. We set off again in search of the house Colonel Bouvet had told us about but there was no sign of it. The Colonel and I therefore left our hated backpacks with the others to bring in and set off to the nearest village which was signposted 5 kilometres away.

When we reached the outskirts of the village we discovered that it was the same village that we had landed at – Le Canadel, now cleared of Germans. We walked down to the beach to find out what had happened to David Rowlands and Nocetto and the panniers. We were afraid they might have been annihilated by the US Air Force. To our delight, and theirs, we found them still intact sheltering in a small station near the beach. In spite of both being slightly wounded, Nocetto with several holes in his tin hat, they were in good heart and the panniers were as we had left them.

They had set up a first-aid post and treated several civilians. They thought we must have been killed or taken prisoner and had decided to give us another hour before moving away from the beach and into a house in the village. Joan and I rushed into the sea to bathe our blistered feet and try to wash some of the grime off our faces and limbs before joining the others in search of a suitable house.

The village of Le Canadel had been badly bombed by the Americans. There were gaping holes in the road and some of the houses had been wrecked. The few inhabitants we met were in a daze from what had happened to them; notwithstanding, they came to our aid when we explained who we were. We told them that we must find a house immediately in which to set up our first-aid post. They suggested the house belonging to the mayor, which was one of the largest in the village, as he was also a well known collaborator with the Germans and a Vichyist.

The Colonel marched up to the mayor's house and informed him and his wife that he was requisitioning their house. They could remain if they wished but were not to interfere with us and we required all but two of their rooms. They were an elderly couple and decided to remain. They were unsympathetic towards us and made no attempt to assist, so we took whatever we needed, including the sheets and the beds in the room Joan and I slept in, which made the old woman particularly angry. We might have felt sorry for them if they had been more helpful. The windows had been blown in and there was glass and dust everywhere, the furniture and china ornaments broken and the mayor and his wife pushed into a corner of their own house with strange people taking it over. They showed no pity towards the wounded, not even giving the patients a drink of water when they were waiting outside on their stretchers.

The wounded were mostly German and American military and some civilians. The Colonel and David Rowlands went off to do an urgent amputation so Joan and I swept up the broken glass as best we could and then pushed most of the furniture into the garden. We turned a small study into an operating theatre and the drawing room and dining room into wards.

When we had cleaned up all the débris we got all the wounded into the house, unpacked the medical supplies and gave plasma to those who needed it, examined their wounds and arranged them in order for operation. A Frenchman and his two teenage daughters arrived, offering to help. We asked them to take over the kitchen and make drinks for the wounded and find whatever food they could for us in the village until the rations arrived.

Two women with wounds on their feet were brought to us by a German sergeant, a Red Cross orderly who volunteered to help us in any way he could. By the time the Colonel returned we had 40 patients. The Colonel had been unable to save the life of the man he had operated on in the village and he immediately started to operate on the ones we had collected.

There was no electricity or water in the house. All the water we needed had to be carried in buckets from a small mountain spring, half way up the hill behind the house. The civilians organised this for us. For an operating table we balanced the stretchers on the backs of two kitchen chairs and Joan and I took it in turns to hold a heavy electric torch over the site to be operated on. Keeping it steady was exhausting work and our arms ached.

While one of us was doing this the other continued to give transfusions of plasma, changed dressings, checked the latest arrivals and kept an eye on the patients recovering from their anaesthetics. David Rowlands had his precious steriliser working at full blast and was busy cleaning and sterilising the instruments as soon as the Colonel finished each operation. Mergier was assisting the Colonel, Jibery gave the anaesthetics and Nocetto kept the record of all the patients and dealt with the rations (when these eventually arrived). It all worked like clockwork and the German sergeant was everywhere giving help to us all.

There was a lull at midnight and the Colonel sent Jean and me up to our room for a rest. Hardly had we shut our eyes when we were called up again as more wounded arrived. The Colonel started operating again and finished at 6am when we all snatched two hours sleep, leaving the wounded in the charge of the two young French girls and the German. We were all pretty dead-beat.

A few guns continued to fire all night and the odd plane flew over but no bombs were dropped. In the early morning we heard the rumble of tanks on the road below us and knew that the rest of the invasion force was arriving.

16 August – While Joan and I were cleaning up the operating theatre from the night before a Captain from the Commandos arrived with the news and much needed rations for the wounded and ourselves. He told us, among other things, that we had been extremely lucky to have been landed on the wrong beach at Le Canadel. Our intended beach at Tayol was heavily mined whereas Le Canadel was so small that the Germans never imagined it would be used for a landing and had kept it as a private beach for themselves.

The Commandos also sent us German medical supplies, which we badly needed as we were running out of ether and dressings. We were surprised at the poor quality: paper bandages, paper gauze and unrefined, non-absorbent cotton wool. Our rations were German as well and pretty nasty. Tinned stew (mostly barley), ersatz coffee and hard black bread. Our French cooks did the best they could by adding all sorts of herbs with fresh vegetables, when they could find some, as well as cheap red wine, of which there was plenty.

The Commandos sent us four Armenian prisoners in the charge of a German Captain to help with the work. The local French had asked us to have the Captain because he had been kind to the local population. He wasn't much use to us and spent most of his time shut up in the room we had given him at the top of the house. The Armenians were not much better as orderlies; the only wounded they would do anything for were six Armenians, all light cases. So we put them in charge of the six horses and three carts we had been given as transport and sent them off to collect rations and supplies and to transfer the wounded civilians to civilian hospitals.

We had no guards for the prisoners and realised afterwards that they could easily have blown us up, or shot us, with the equipment strewn all over the place belonging to the wounded (rifles, revolvers, hand grenades and Sten guns) during the first hectic hours when no one had time to sort it out.

The only prisoner of any worth that we had collected was our volunteer German sergeant. He was a Prussian, tall, fair and very good looking. He could speak a little French and told us his name was Poppi. He was worth all the others put together and worked every bit as hard as we did and had the initiative to do jobs that needed doing without being told. He organised the unwilling Armenians and made them dig latrines in the garden. He collected all the armaments and stacked them in the garden shed and found a padlock to secure the door. He was always in a good temper and accepted, with a smile, any job we asked him to do. He was kind and gentle to the wounded, looking after them with devotion and, unlike the Armenians, treating all the patients equally, making no distinction between German, French or American. We tried hard to keep him with us for as long as we were with the Commandos but he was taken away from us when we left Le Lavandou, our next stopping place. I often wondered what happened to him.

During the day the Colonel sent Jibery and Joan off in one of the carts to contact Commando HQ and find out if there were any instructions for us. There were – we were to move nearer to the front. I stayed on duty until 3am and then handed over to Poppi and the French girls who had all had a rest. Joan (who was even more tired than I was) and I slept like logs until morning, the longest sleep we'd had since we left the *Prince David*.

Next morning we started evacuating the wounded in our carts to the nearest civilian hospital, but as soon as they left they were replaced by others and we were kept busy day and night. Whenever one of us had a spare moment we popped to the kitchen to help with the cooking for the patients and grab something for ourselves, and we drank endless cups of coffee to keep us awake.

Colonel Lotte, the Divisional Medical Officer, paid us a visit in the afternoon with Commandant St Hilier, Chief of Staff to General Brosset, to find out how we were faring and to tell us that the division had arrived. A Commando liaison officer arrived to collect the Colonel and find a new site for us. The Colonel returned with the news that he had found a large hotel overlooking the sea at Le Lavandou, about five kilometres away, and we would move there next day after lunch.

18 August – All the patients, except four seriously wounded ones, were evacuated and no more arrived. As soon as the last one had left we packed everything up, loaded it all into the three carts and sent them off to Le Lavandou. Joan and I found time to rush down to the sea and have a bathe and, after a quick lunch, we climbed on top of a large antiquated lorry piled high with bales of hay and sacks of corn for our horses. There were the seven of us plus the two French girls, Silvie and Claude, and Poppi. Our patients followed in an American ambulance which Colonel Lotte had borrowed for us. Off we bumped along the five kilometres to Le Lavandou, one of the strangest convoys of the war.

The Germans had used the hotel at Le Lavandou as a barracks, and had left it in a filthy condition. All the lavatories were broken and blocked and smeared with human excreta. Everywhere else was in the same disgusting state and, of course, there was no water or electricity. At least there was plenty of space, as the hotel was three storeys high and there was room for everyone to be housed inside. Joan and I found a bedroom on the third floor which was comparatively clean and completely empty except for a portable bidet, which made us laugh. We took two stretchers for beds and used our greatcoats as blankets but it was so hot we seldom used them. Having dumped our packs in our room we set about cleaning the rooms downstairs and unpacking all the equipment again. A large reception room capable of holding four rows of stretchers served as the main ward. Several smaller rooms led out of it. One served as an operating theatre and another as a resuscitation ward; the remainder came into use as wards when the main one overflowed.

We found a long table which we put at one end of the ward and stacked our dressings and instruments on it. Someone brought two enormous rubber containers on iron stands with four taps at their bottom for water, which we put outside on the balcony. They looked exactly like an outsize cow's udders.

We hadn't finished unpacking before a queue of civilians formed, all with minor wounds to be dressed. They were followed by Commando wounded. The Colonel operated on one urgent abdominal case and decided to leave the rest until the morning. He told us to get as much sleep as we could, so Joan and I divided the night between us, each getting about five hours' sleep.

Our first two civilian volunteers arrived early next morning and were a curious contrast: the midwife of Le Lavandou and the local tart. The midwife, Madame Anne, was a small elderly lady with snow-white hair, bright blue eyes and a face as round as an apple. The town's prostitute (so we were told later), Lily, had violent red hair and a green satin skirt above her knees, topped by a white apron and very high-heeled shoes. They were both invaluable and I don't think we would have coped without their help. Madame Anne took over all the cooking, providing hot meals for all the patients and us. Lily, indefatigable, tripped up and down the ward on her high-heeled shoes, gave drinks, arranged pillows, helped with the meals and, through her many contacts, provided us with all we needed. We only had to ask and it appeared – eau de cologne and talcum powder for backs, trays for meals, and all sorts of little extras for the patients.

The Resistance organised lorries to collect beds, mattresses, pillows, sheets, blankets, tables, chairs, china, cutlery, every necessity, all generously provided by the inhabitants of Le Lavandou for our hospital. Fruit, vegetables, bread, wine and mineral water were brought daily to the kitchen. The local women undertook to wash the dirty linen and clean the wards, and helped Madame Anne with the cooking and washing up. Whenever a soldier died, whatever his nationality, the entire town arranged and attended his funeral in the little church and graveyard.

The only helpers who bothered us were the civilian doctors, who tried to take over from Joan and me, coming into the wards uninvited and ignorant of the routine we had established. They undid dressings we had already done or did others without our knowledge. They took our instruments, wasted our dressings and only hindered us whatever their good intentions were. The Colonel had to ask them to leave us alone. We collected two skilled nurses out of the many volunteers. One man relieved us of much anxiety by looking after the delirious patients and the frequently violent head cases. The other, a Belgian sister called Simone, whose standard of nursing was equal to the best, took over as night sister when there were no operations which meant Joan and I could get some sleep at night.

We learnt that three-quarters of the division had disembarked and, with the Commandos, was to go into action to liberate Toulon where there was a strong force of Germans. Apparently the Hadfield–Spears Hospital would not be arriving for several days which meant that we would have to look after the divisional wounded as well as the Commandos.

By the evening, the main ward was full as was the balcony running alongside it, and all the downstairs rooms. Our patients were Commandos, Americans, Germans, civilians and a few men from the Division. The Colonel continued to operate until 10pm and two soldiers died.

20 August – Two French women who had collaborated with the Germans were brought into the hotel under guard to scrub floors. The mayor of Le Lavandou, followed by a procession of the town's dignitaries, arrived with them and they were led through while the mayor made a speech describing their wrong-doings to the wounded, who appeared to be as embarrassed as we were. The women's hair had been shaved off except for a tuft at the top of their heads. Their guard, a fierce looking Maquis with a home-made Sten gun, kept poking them in the ribs if they did not work fast enough to satisfy him. The younger of the two women was later vindicated; she was one of the inmates of the local brothel and obviously could not choose her clients. They could not give her back her hair, but she covered her head with a scarf and implored us to let her remain and continue work for us as she said we were the only people who had been kind to her. She was a marvellous worker and whenever possible took the disagreeable jobs that the other woman avoided.

No more wounded arrived that morning but the operations continued on the wounded from the day before. The Colonel gave Joan and me the morning off. Joan went for a swim on the beach below the hotel; then wandered round Le Lavandou. She said there wasn't much to see and no shops. I had had my eye on one of the Armenians' horses; it was obviously a cut above the others and looked like an officer's charger. A stallion, grey-white in colour, probably an Arab. He had his own saddle and bridle so I got on him and went for a ride up into the hills following a lane, then took footpaths through the trees. He was beautifully schooled and had the comfortable trot of an Arab horse so that the rider hardly moves in the saddle. I passed a few isolated houses hidden in the wood and imagined that they were foresters' houses. There seemed to be no animals or birds but it was so peaceful and marvellous to escape for a few hours from the horror of the wounded and dying soldiers and from the hospital, able to be on my own on a beautiful horse riding through a pretty forest.

The hospital was comparatively quiet all that day with no admissions and at 8pm we were wondering how soon we would be able to finish our work, leave Simone in charge, and go to bed when an ambulance arrived followed by another, and another, and yet another. 112 wounded were admitted by midnight which, with the 100 or so we already had, swelled the numbers to well over 200.

It was like a nightmare. I kept repeating to myself: 'This can't continue'. Stretchers filled the passages, the balconies and all the small rooms on the second and third floors. Luckily for us – and for them – not all the wounded were serious cases. I'll never forget Joan and me groping our way through rows and rows of stretchers holding a flickering German torch in one hand and a pair of scissors in the other. We were looking for the most seriously wounded and at the same time keeping three or four plasma drips running. We also had to shave the heads of several badly smashed skulls with a cut-throat razor in the light of a flickering candle before sending them through to the theatre.

Some of the wounded were so badly injured that we could do nothing for them except administer morphia. One thing that struck me forcibly, and often, was the difference in attitude regarding the will to live. There is no doubt at all that determination to survive, or lack of it, played a greater part in their recovery (or death) than anything we could do for patients. One could never tell from the injuries alone who would pull through and who would not.

The most miraculous recovery I ever witnessed was made by a légionnaire who was brought in during the night with multiple injuries. He had been blown up by a land mine while rescuing his officer, who had been shot in the stomach and was seriously wounded. They both arrived in the same ambulance. The légionnaire had both legs shattered below the knees, and a gaping wound in his chest from which bubbled a mixture of froth and blood as he breathed. He had another wound in his back from which he was haemorrhaging; a large piece of shrapnel was sticking out which had pierced a kidney. He was completely conscious. I gave him two plasma transfusions and sent him off to theatre. The Colonel sent him back again with a message to say that this case was hopeless and that he must conserve his time for the wounded who had a chance of survival. The légionnaire's courage in rescuing his officer from the minefield, and his uncomplaining acceptance of his wounds, made me determined to try and save his life if I could. I made a gentleman's agreement with the Colonel that if the légionnaire was still alive in the morning I could send him back to theatre and we would do what he could for him.

I gave him several more transfusions of plasma during the night but he continued to haemorrhage from his wounds and passed large amounts of blood in his urine. I wasn't very hopeful. Next morning, however, he was still alive and fully conscious. The Colonel grudgingly agreed to operate on him, but only after he had finished his main list. This he did after I had given my patient one more transfusion at about midday. The légionnaire returned from the theatre with both legs in plaster, although the Colonel thought he would have to have them amputated later – if he survived. A tube was in his chest, which was no longer bubbling air and blood, the shrapnel had been removed and one of his kidneys had been taken out and the other stitched up. He was still alive and making good progress when we moved on from Le Lavandou a few days later. He had to have one leg amputated at the hospital he was evacuated to; the other was saved and he recovered. I am convinced that it was his will to live that saved him. I was furious with the officer whom he had saved from the minefield. His wife came every day to visit him with fruit and cakes and never offered anything to the légionnaire. In the end I went to him and said: 'Don't you think you could give something to the soldier who saved your life?'

21 August – The Colonel continued to operate all day. We rushed from patient to patient, changing dressings and looking after them as best we could. Several of the wounded died which, alas, was inevitable. Joan and I divided the wards up between us. She took over the side wards and balconies and I remained in the main ward.

Some time during the morning when I was at the bottom of the ward away from the entrance and in the middle of changing blood-hardened dressings of a double leg amputation, which always takes time and is excruciatingly painful for the patient, in spite of the help of a large injection of morphia, I saw out of the corner of my eye a man in a blue blouse with the Resistance brassard on his arm and four young boys enter the room and stand by the dressing table, at the top of the ward, looking rather embarrassed. 'Hell,' I thought,'If I've got to look after civilians as well it's too much.' I decided that they would have to wait until I had finished the dressing on my patient. I guessed they could not be all that badly wounded if they had walked in.

When I had finished I picked up my tray of dirty dressings and instruments and slowly made my way along the ward to where they were standing. On reaching them I saw, to my horror, that they were burnt from head to foot. They continued to stand mutely while I stood like a stone staring straight at them. All their hair, eyebrows and lashes were burnt away. Their faces, arms and chests were a deathly white with flakes of skin hanging from them. Two of them had leather belts burnt into their waists. They were completely naked except for their pants, and had blankets over their shoulders. The smell of burnt flesh was sickening.

For the first and, I think, the only time in my life I forgot my hospital training and panicked. I rushed into the operating theatre and shouted for the Colonel to come at once. He was so surprised that he dropped his instruments and came. He took one look at the boys and, taking me to one side said: 'Morphia. We can't do anything else'. I said: 'Nothing?' and he replied: 'Give them as much morphia as you like. They will all die.' I couldn't believe it. I moved four of the less severely wounded out of their beds and on to stretchers, put the boys between clean sheets in the beds and gave them all double doses of morphia.

The man who brought them in told me their story. The eldest boy was nineteen, the youngest fifteen. They had volunteered to guide the Resistance to a spot under the hills where they had watched the Germans bury a quantity of petrol. What they did not know was that the Germans had ringed the site with mines. One boy was killed outright. He had stepped on a mine which had exploded and ignited the petrol which engulfed the others. They had walked two miles to the hospital, completely naked except for their underpants, which were only scorched. It was only when they reached the hospital that they had been given blankets by Nocetta who had no idea of the seriousness of their condition.

The fifteen-year-old boy was the brother of one of the girls helping us at the hospital and was slightly less badly burnt than the others. I tried to save his life. I found a small area on each of his thighs which had not been burnt and succeeded in getting a needle into each of the veins in these areas and gave him a continuous plasma drip. I got his sister to stay beside him and told her that if he could pass urine it would be a helpful sign. Every hour she gave him the urinal and pleaded with him to try. The poor boy became more and more anxious as he was unable to produce a drop, and her anxiety increased as well. I also told her to get him to drink as much as he could, but this did not help. I cut down his morphia as much as I could and kept up the transfusions but he died just the same. I wished that I had not prolonged the agony by helping him to live for three extra days. The other three boys had died within 36 hours.

Nursing these boys was terrible. We propped them up with pillows as they had great difficulty in breathing and kept slipping down their beds. Every time we lifted them up pieces of their skin were left on our arms and the smell of burnt flesh clung to our bodies and clothes. We made cradles from cardboard boxes to put over them to keep the weight of the bed clothes away from their poor burnt bodies and tried to cover the worst of their burns with pieces of gauze soaked in sterile liquid paraffin.

These boys continued to haunt me and will continue to do so for the rest of my life. They were so young and brave, and they never complained.

The last three days we spent at Le Lavandou were not so hectic and Joan and I were able to snatch an hour or two off duty. I rode my white charger through the forest and was able to forget for a while the wounded at the hospital. On the last day I was cantering along my usual lane and past one of the houses in the forest when I came upon a funeral procession about to start. To my horror I recognised the sister and parents of the boy whose life I had tried so desperately to save. I felt awful, enjoying my ride while they were mourning their son. I was covered in shame.

22 August – We evacuated all the movable wounded, keeping only les grands blessés, and although we continued to have a steady trickle of wounded we never again had an influx comparable to the night of the twentieth. Each day we became better organised, with the voluntary helpers each assigned to particular jobs and knowing what to do. This meant that we could snatch the odd hour off duty for a quick bathe in the sea or, for me, a ride on my white charger.

The Commandos had given the Colonel a civilian Ford car, which was a great improvement on the horses and ramshackle old lorry we had used until now. I began to drive again as well as nurse – a welcome change. The Colonel tried to get to Toulon by himself to see how the fighting was progressing but never reached the town as it was still in the hands of the Germans. He had six punctures on the way there and three on the return trip as the tyres were badly worn. The rumour that we were to continue with the spearhead of the division as its forward medical unit turned out to be true – engineered by the Colonel, I have no doubt, whose sense of adventure surpassed that of most other people.

A Red Cross commandant arrived in the hospital one morning, the Comtesse someone or other. She immediately started to try and organise us and the running of the hospital. She informed us that Lily was the local prostitute (which we already knew) and must be sent away at once. This made me lose my temper and I told her we did not need her. Luckily for me the Colonel arrived at that moment and agreed with me. He told her that as long as we ran the hospital Lily stayed. The Comtesse someone or other left in disgust. Like many others, she had only come near us when it was obvious that we were there to stay, unlike Lily and Madame Anne who had offered us their help from the very beginning.

We left Le Lavandou on 3 August, handing over the hospital with all its patients to the civilian doctors and authorities, but taking with us our replenished panniers and the precious steriliser. Lily, Sylvie, Simone and Claude all wanted to come with us but we were not allowed to take them – nor Poppi who, alas, was sent to a prisoner-of-war camp. The horses and carts were also left behind as we now had a Commando jeep as well as the Colonel's Ford, which was sufficient transport for the seven of us and our equipment.

To recap on our work at Le Lavandou we admitted 345 wounded, 50 of them from the Commandos, 180 from our division of the Free French and 80 from other French units, 6 Americans, 8 civilians and 18 Germans. As well as these we had numerous lightly wounded whose wounds we dressed before returning them to their units, homes, civilian hospitals or prisoner-of-war camps.

12

FORWARD UNIT TO LYONS

We set off from Le Lavandou for Hyères in a Renault CV which the Commandos had given us. Hyères, a small town some 20 miles from Toulon, had been liberated on the twentieth. Our destination was the civilian hospital, which the Colonel had been ordered to clean up and turn into a base hospital for the division.

Our reception at the hospital was cold to say the least. In the main hall were large posters of Pétain and of a Vichy rally calling the youth of France to arms in the German legion. We took great pleasure in tearing them down under the disapproving eyes of the matron and senior medical officer. The matron took us on a round of the wards and theatre which were staffed by nuns and slatternly nurses in dirty uniforms. The wards were filthy, the bed linen soiled and the dressings looked as if they had not been changed for days. The atmosphere of the hospital staff was decidedly antagonistic towards us – almost sinister – and neither Joan nor I fancied working there. The Colonel raised hell and had the entire staff assembled in the hall and told them he would give them 24 hours – no more – to get the wards and theatre cleaned up. There were angry squeaks of indignation and many excuses.

Having delivered his rocket the Colonel drove us all back to Le Canadel for a bathe in the sea. We had two punctures on the way there. Several of the villagers recognised us and gave us presents of eggs, white bread and butter. This was just as well as the matron at Hyères said she had no rations for us, so we got in the car again and made a picnic of our gifts. The matron turned two of her nurses out of their bedroom for Joan and me, which did not increase our popularity – specially when we demanded clean sheets and bedding, which were grudgingly given to us.

There was no water or electricity in the hospital which had originally been a hotel. All the wash basins were blocked up as were the two lavatories for both staff and patients, their seats side by side in a shed in the garden, with no proper door or lock, one bucket of water between the two and as filthy as the rest of the place. We had been much better off than this at Le Canadel and Le Lavandou.

24 August – A definite change for the better in the attitude of the hospital staff towards us, perhaps because the Colonel told Joan and me that we were not to do any work in the hospital except to

accompany him on his ward rounds. We had lunch with the staff: black bread, and lukewarm soup with bits of suspicious-looking meat floating on it. Grey lentils and grey coffee with saccharine. No wonder the nurses were so sour and bad tempered.

We escaped after this sad meal and, back to my real job as a driver, I drove the Colonel, Nocetto and Joan to Toulon with Nocetto, whose wife and family lived nearby, pointing out places of interest along the route. We saw many examples of German destruction and paid a visit to Nocetto's aunt and uncle, who were very friendly and regaled us with stories of German brutality.

The kindness of the local people never ceased to surprise me. We met none of this from the Italians, in spite of the fact that many of our patients were Italian civilians and we had brought them peace. Perhaps they were still too frightened and apprehensive. The French, although they had very little themselves, loaded us with food and invitations to meals. They offered us help in any way they could in the hospital. The poorer they were, the more generous they were, or so it appeared to me. Only the staff at the hospital at Hyères were unfriendly.

We visited several units of the division on our trip and heard the latest details of the fight for Toulon, which was virtually over. As we approached the outskirts of Toulon there was plenty of evidence of the battle – houses burning, soldiers fighting their way through crowds of civilians into buildings, the rat-tat-tat of machine gun fire and corpses of horses and humans littering the streets. Vehicles and débris blocked the streets and people wandered around with dazed expressions on their faces. On our return journey we drove by the coast road and through a village called Les Deux Oiseaux to an empty, mined and booby-trapped laundry which the Colonel thought might serve as a hospital for us once it had been cleared, but we had to turn it down as it was in too bad a condition. Sylvie, Claude and Simone were waiting for us when we returned to Hyères and we all went off from the girls' villa in Le Canadel to bathe. Later we found some white bread in a bakery and all had a picnic supper.

Paris was liberated on 25 August and the Colonel decided to celebrate the occasion at Hyères the next day. I drove off in a borrowed army pick-up to Divisional HQ to collect a bugler and Croix de Lorraine flag. The entire hospital watched the raising of this flag.

We were doing no work now because Toulon had fallen to the division, and the Naval hospital being on the spot, so to speak, fully equipped and staffed, received the divisional wounded until the front moved further away and Spears Hospital arrived.

I returned the bugler and his flag to the HQ, and then drove Joan and David Rowlands to Le Lavandou for our last farewells. While Joan and David went bathing I had the unpleasant task of trying to find a home for the horses; no one wanted them, and their Armenian grooms had been sent to a PoW camp. Finally, I was obliged to give them to the mayor of Le Lavandou, who was also the town's butcher. He promised me he would feed and care for them until he slaughtered them. I thought they deserved a better fate; the officer's charger, which I had enjoyed riding so much, was a beautiful horse and it was awful to think of him being slaughtered.

After this, I joined Joan and David at Le Lavandou. Having said our goodbyes to all the patients and civilian staff, Simone took us to lunch with her uncle and aunt who had prepared a memorable feast for us: *Œuf poché à la Florentine*, roast rabbit with *sauté* potatoes, and rich creamy *entremets*, rare Beaune wine (which they had been keeping for a special occasion), fruit, real coffee and cognac. We could hardly get up from the table at the end of the meal.

Following this marvellous feast, Simone took Joan and me to a hairdresser for a much-needed shampoo; then back to her house for our first bath in soft water since we had landed in France. It was to be a long time before we had another. Simone lent us some clean underclothes and promised to wash our dirty linen for us to pick up the next day.

Back at the hospital we learnt that the matron had arranged a dinner party in our honour but Joan and I had no intention of attending after the way she had treated us. Fortunately, we had accepted an invitation to dine with Captain Montgraham of the Commandos who had been reunited with his family living in a villa on the outskirts of Hyères. Montgraham collected us from the hospital; no sooner had we arrived at his house than the Colonel sent a message to recall us to the hospital immediately. Returning, we were told that we were to leave with the division for the Rhone Valley at 6.30 the next morning as their forward unit.

The Colonel returned with us to the Montgrahams and after dinner drove us over to Simone's house to collect our still-wet washing. The Colonel told Simone that we could not take her with us and we said our sad goodbyes.

27 August – Up at 5am to pack and load up. We reached the division at 6am and were told that they were not moving off until 8 o'clock. The Colonel, always impatient, decided to set off ahead of them, leaving Nocetto with the jeep and equipment to follow with the division.

We drove through Toulon to Marseilles which, except for the docks, was not nearly as badly damaged as Toulon. The countryside between Toulon and Marseilles was very picturesque, hilly and at times mountainous, pine trees on all the hills, great rocks sticking out, and gorges. From Marseilles to Aix it became less mountainous; the farther we went the flatter the landscape became, with more cultivation, orchards and vineyards.

Aix was a very pretty town with a fountain playing in the main square. It had been liberated seven days before and the streets were full of people and American troops. There was a considerable amount of shell fire around Aix and the usual sight of wandering refugees, wounded and dead civilians and Resistance fighters.

We stopped for a drink at the Deux Garçons, a famous bistro in Aix, and then visited a friend of the Colonel's where we were given another enormous spread for lunch: sardines, pâté, white bread, apricots in syrup, wine and real coffee – all produced at a moment's notice. Our meals then were most bizarre and unpredictable – subsistence army rations snatched at odd moments, interspersed with banquets provided by the grateful liberated French.

The division caught us up near St Remy de Provence and we joined them in convoy. The sides of the roads were lined with people clapping their hands, waving flags and throwing flowers and fruit into our vehicles. Melons hurt when they hit you!

We spent the night in a field near a college. Joan and I set off to collect water to wash in and to drink. We had hardly settled down when the Colonel and Commandant Terramorsi of the ACL, who had joined us after we left Hyères, called us back and said they were taking us to Avignon, some 25 kilometres away in Terramorsi's jeep, which I was to drive. Halfway there an elderly cyclist collided with me and bounced into a ditch. We picked him up and dusted him down; he was quite unharmed but very drunk, having celebrated the liberation in every bistro on his way home. We returned him – and his buckled bicycle – to his house before we continued on our way.

We toured Avignon, visiting the famous Pont d'Avignon and the Pope's Palace. The bridge over the river before Avignon had been blown up and we were directed to a ford. I took the fan belt off the jeep as the water came over the bonnet. We managed to get through, helped by crowds of delighted spectators who helped to push us.

An emotional and thickly bearded Frenchman got me in a bear hug shouting: *'Une femme française'*. When I spluttered that I was *'Une Anglaise'* he replied: *'Beaucoup mieux'* and gave me another hug. An embarrassing number of others followed his example, while I struggled to get the fan belt on again.

All the women tried to grab our hands and touch our uniforms, as if they could not believe that we were real. Children were held up and carried over their parents' heads for us to hold or kiss, and endless photographs were taken before we were allowed to continue on our way.

Avignon was draped with French, English and American flags and the crowds were so thick that it was difficult to drive through them without harming anyone. Terramorsi stood up in the back of the jeep shouting: *'Vive de Gaulle'*. Sometimes there were cheers; sometimes none – it seemed that a great number of French people in the South had never heard of de Gaulle.

We returned to our field for our supper of army rations and then all went off to Les Baux. We drove through magnificent scenery and ended up in a bistro perched on top of a gorge. Everyone wanted to shake our hands, and peered at *Les Anglaises* as if we had descended from Mars.

When we entered the bistro, which was full of Frenchmen, there was complete silence. Their hands went to their pockets, and we wondered for a moment whether they were going to shoot us. But as soon as the Colonel shouted: *'Français, Français libre, et de Gaulle'* we received the friendliest of welcomes.

28 August – We were summoned to the divisional HQ and asked if we would volunteer to accompany a spearhead of divisional shock troops consisting of the Fusiliers Marins and the Foreign Legion, whose orders were to harry and harass the German retreat up the Rhône Valley on the right-hand side of the river. The remainder of the division would be regrouped after their brief and bloody effort in liberating Toulon and Marseilles to conserve their meagre supply of petrol.

Without asking us, the Colonel accepted without a moment's hesitation. We would be called *Le Service Chirurgical d'Urgence* (Emergency Surgical Service) and our transport would be provided for us by the Compagnie de Ramassage No 3 under the command of our good friend Terramorsi, who would leave his unit, the ACL. We were given six ambulances as well as pick-ups and jeeps, which ensured our ability to keep up with the shock troops wherever they were.

The ACL and the remainder of Terramorsi's fleet of ambulances were furious that we had been chosen, arguing that we had had our share of excitement when we landed with the Commandos. The Colonel pointed out, with good reason, that we were the only ones with the necessary experience of improvisation and had already proved that we were an efficient team.

We waved goodbye to the division at 5 o'clock next morning and, together with Terramorsi and his ambulances and trucks, made our way by lanes and secondary roads to the Rhône crossing.

We reached our destination at 7pm, before either the Fusilier Marins or the Foreign Legion, and before anyone realised what was happening. The Colonel in his car, and Terramorsi in one of his ambulances, had driven on to the makeshift ferry – to the surprise of the group of Sappers who had built it. When they had recovered, they tried to get us off again, but nothing would budge the Colonel. Then the Legion arrived and furiously told the Colonel to get his vehicles off the ferry, indignantly demanding what would he do if he met the Germans on his own. No argument would move the Colonel, and the Heath Robinson ferry – consisting of six or eight small boats, four with outboard motors, lashed together with ropes and planks of wood laid across them for vehicles to drive on to – started drifting across the river.

The crossing was a zig-zag performance. The current of the river was very strong and halfway across two of the four engines cut out. It was then that the Sapper officer in charge told us that they had not been at all certain that the ferry would work. They had intended to do a trial run unloaded but, as we had plonked ourselves on board, it would have been difficult, if not impossible, to reverse us off again so they decided to risk it. We reached the other side of the river eventually, much lower down than intended, and it took the Sappers some time to make us secure and put down more planks so that we could drive off the ferry and up the bank.

We parked ourselves in a field off the roadside surrounded by vines, tomatoes and peach trees. We put up our hospital sign by the side of the road so that the others could find us. I walked across the field to a small farmhouse and knocked on the door. It was opened by a woman who told me that she was Polish. I asked her if she could give me some hot water for our Nescafé. She insisted that I went back to fetch the others and that we must all come to her kitchen to heat our rations on her stove. She gave us tomatoes and fruit to eat and some rough red wine to drink.

After our meal the four of us set off for some more sightseeing. Firstly we went to Pont du Gard and were relieved to find the Roman aqueduct still intact. Later we learnt that the Germans had mined it and that the Maquis had defused all the mines the same night.

Nîmes was our next destination but by the time we arrived it was late and the town was in utter darkness. The Colonel took us to look at the school he had attended as a boy and to the hospital where he had done his medical training. We then went to the coliseum and other Roman remains. To our surprise the few people in the streets gave us sullen looks. We found a bistro which looked more or less open and pushed our way inside. We were served by a sour looking proprietor. It wasn't until we started questioning a group of Frenchmen, who had surrounded our table and had been glaring at us with menacing faces, that we discovered that we were the first Allied personnel to enter Nîmes. In the dark they thought we were the advance guard of the German column. They told us we were lucky not to have been shot at or blown up. When they realised who we were their enthusiasm became embarrassing. They asked us endless questions as more and more Frenchmen arrived to inspect us and eventually the Colonel decided that our only course was a quick getaway back to our field in case the Germans really did turn up.

29 August – We had to sleep on the ground without mosquito nets and were nearly bitten to death during the night. The Polish lady came across early in the morning to tell us that she had prepared breakfast for us all in her house. What a breakfast! *Café au lait* in huge bowls, two fried eggs each, and freshly baked bread and butter. She shyly said she had been told by her mother that *Les Anglaises* always ate eggs for breakfast.

The kindness and generosity of the poorer French people towards us never ceased to astonish me. The farmer and his wife were living a breadline existence with a few ducks and chickens, a cow, a goat and a few rabbits. They cultivated fruit and vegetables and sold them in the market. They had three small children who looked half-starved and were poorly clad. Their poverty did not prevent them from killing one of their rabbits and insisting that we had our evening meal with them.

After breakfast we went with the Colonel to choose a site for our hospital near Pont du Gard. We found what was once a luxury hotel overlooking the river. It had been left in the usual state of indescribable filth by the Germans. Every room had been stripped of all movable furniture, the remainder was deliberately smashed. Urine and excrement were everywhere, even smeared on the walls. They had driven a pick axe into the boiler, the lavatories were either broken or overflowing with excreta all over the walls and floors. The smell was asphyxiating.

In one room downstairs we found some putrefying German corpses and in another room three badly wounded German soldiers in a pitiable condition. The Colonel was beside himself with rage and sent for thirty German prisoners to clean the whole place up.

By midday sufficient rooms had been cleaned to be used as wards. We moved the three Germans into a ward where we dressed their wounds and washed and fed them. As usual, there was no water or electricity. We found a well in the courtyard which was in working order and unpolluted. We broke into a locked shed and found shelves of medical equipment, boxes of plaster bandages and supplies – a bonus, as we were very low on these items.

In the afternoon, as no patients had arrived, we returned to Nîmes to see it in daylight. It was a different place from the night before; full of jubilant crowds who mobbed us. A few shops were open and we were showered with gifts from them and not allowed to pay for anything.

We returned to our field to collect our belongings, and the painful task of explaining to our Polish friend that we couldn't stay for supper as we had to return to Pont du Gard in case any wounded had arrived. She already had pots cooking on her stove but, quite undaunted, she sent her husband off to kill another rabbit and, in spite of our protests, insisted that we take it and cook it ourselves. While her husband was preparing the rabbit she filled the jeep with fruit and two bottles of wine.

By the time we returned to the hospital several wounded had been delivered including five grands blessés who were hospitalised. The rest were treated and returned to their units or evacuated to a civilian hospital.

We were told that 'Spears' had at last disembarked at St Raphael and were on their way to join the division. The Colonel rushed off to find them and we cooked our rabbit in a tin basin we found over a wood fire. It tasted quite good – better than bully beef or spam.

30 August – The Colonel returned in a very bad temper; he had driven all night, failed to find Spears, and had smashed up his car by falling asleep and wrapping it around a tree. He was none the worse, but his car was. Terramorsi and I drove it into Nîmes and found a garage whose owner repaired it while we waited. He refused to be paid for the work, and told us he could get us a brand new car for nothing if we were still there in two or three days – which, alas, we were not.

No more patients arrived and in the afternoon the Colonel took us in his repaired car to visit an enchanted château nearby. It was hidden among leafy trees and was very old and built of grey stone. Great wrought iron gates opened to a short drive. A brass-studded door led to an immense banqueting hall, the walls of which were panelled with triumphant battle scenes. Leading from the hall was a series of reception rooms, some panelled in wood, others with paintings, frescoes, or rich brocade hangings. A stone staircase with a beautifully decorated wrought iron hand-rail curled round the outside of the chateau, leading to the first and second floors. The bedrooms were furnished with delicate eighteenth-century furniture. Everywhere there was evidence of a hasty retreat by the Germans, which was probably why nothing had been destroyed. Bureau drawers hung open, chairs were upturned, beds unmade and there were papers everywhere.

The château had obviously been used as a headquarters. We found Generals' hats, uniforms, medals, and even dress swords lying around. A half-eaten meal remained on the dining room table with more upturned chairs and wine glasses. We helped ourselves to some of the left-overs and found more bottles of wine, tins of food and supplies in the kitchen. We loaded these into the car.

I went into the courtyard and found a path which led to some wooden army huts. I walked through several barrack rooms and then came to a locked door. I managed to lever the door open with a bayonet which I found lying on one of the beds and found myself in an office which contained, amongst the office equipment, stacks and shelves of maps. They were all of France, three-quarters of an inch to a kilometre. I collected a complete set for myself together with a key map which served me well for the rest of the war. I then rejoined the others and told the Colonel of my find and took him there. We discovered other papers covered with mysterious squares, circles and other marks. The Colonel thought they could be important and sent a scout off to the Deuxième Bureau. A captain and lieutenant arrived at the château and on seeing the maps became very excited, saying that they were of great importance. The mysterious circles and squares were code identification of the German signalling. They also found maps and papers of the latest German battle orders and battle formation. The officers could not understand why the huts had not been booby trapped or mined. I suspected that the Germans simply had not had time to do this any more than they had been able to finish their meal or packing, or to take the information with them.

General Brosset ticked me off about if afterwards and said we were not to go exploring like that on our own again. But he also thanked me and said how lucky it was that I had found them.

When we returned to the hospital after this adventure we found orders waiting for us to move on to Lussan in the Ardèche, some 25 kilometres away. Our wounded had already been evacuated so it didn't take us long to pack up and we were on the road by 4pm.

On our way we came across a bad accident involving men of the Bataillon de Marche, from our division, who had been blown up by a mine buried in the road. We bandaged up all but two who were badly wounded, and sent them on their way. We put the two stretcher cases in one of our ambulances and took them with us.

Lussan was a small medieval village perched on top of a hill and completely surrounded by a wall. We found a suitable empty house, put our sign up outside, and set about cleaning it out and preparing a room for the theatre and another for the ward. The Colonel operated on the two soldiers and we settled them down for the night. To our surprise this house had electricity which worked and plenty of water, which we obtained by winding up a bucket from a deep well in the garden. We cooked ourselves a nice hot meal on an electric stove, which was a pleasant change. While we were in the middle of enjoying the meal thirteen wounded were brought in, all légionnaires. Only one was seriously wounded and he sadly died during the night.

31 August – We kept our patients until midday and then evacuated them. When they had left we set off in Terramorsi's jeep to visit Uzes where we wandered round admiring the old grey stone houses and cobbled streets. We returned to Lussan for tea and found fresh orders instructing us to move to Vallon for the night. The Colonel went off alone to find a site, and while the rest of our party packed up Joan and I made them an English tea of hot buttered toast, jam and cocoa.

The Colonel returned in the evening to say he had found a warm empty barn which would do us very well. Unfortunately, by the time we got there the Foreign Legion had already taken possession and we had to spend the night in an empty, dirty hospital nearby. Next morning we set off early for Tence, 150 kilometres away. The Colonel, Jibery, Joan and I went ahead of our convoy and by a different route hoping to find the Colonel's family, whom he had not seen for six years. We drove through one of the loveliest regions of France starting off along a small road which followed the winding course of a river. The country gradually changed to mountainous ranges, with valleys between and twisty passes through and over them, and swift running streams and rivers between them. Villages and towns were hidden in the valleys and sometimes were perched on top of the mountains as in Italy. The mountains and hilly countryside slowly fell away and green pastures bordered by woods took their place. We passed herds of cattle and flocks of sheep, each guarded by an old woman, always dressed in black and busily knitting – or by young boys playing with sheep dogs.

We stopped to eat our lunch beside a wood nestling under a low hill, supplementing our rations with wild strawberries and raspberries which we found growing under the trees, hidden between the harebells, foxgloves, bilberries and bracken. Apple and chestnut trees laden with fruit lined the roadsides and everywhere looked peaceful and far removed from war.

After many enquiries and wrong turnings we finally ran the Colonel's family to ground at Le Chambon. They were living in a small school house hidden in pine trees. His mother, father, brother, sister-in-law and two of his four children were there when we arrived. It was a tearful and joyful reunion. The Colonel's youngest son, Hervé, had gone down to the nearest town with his school mates to wave to the army convoys driving by. We went in search of him and found him among a crowd of other children. When he saw his father, whom he did not recognise or remember, he became delirious with excitement shouting: '*C'est mon Papa*' and insisted that we drove him around the town so that he could show off his father in the uniform of the Free French. We stayed with the Colonel's family for tea and then left with promises to return.

At Tence we found Terramorsi had installed the unit in a monastery. It was very clean, and once the monks had recovered from the shock of having two women dumped on them – and Protestants at that, as was the Colonel – they were charming and hospitable to us. They put up two beds, with clean linen, for Joan and me in the part of the monastery which had been a school, and gave us the run of their well-equipped kitchen where Joan and I cooked a meal for everyone from our rations and the Abbot gave us some sweet old wine to drink. After supper the Abbot showed Joan and me to a bathroom which had hot running water. We had a much needed bath and washed our hair and underclothes which were all pretty grubby by now.

Next morning the Colonel borrowed Terramorsi's jeep and made a return visit to his family. He drove them across country and while traversing a ditch bumped the head of one of the children against the windscreen and knocked him out. Another child received a black eye when the jeep hit the opposite bank with a bang.

2 September – Early in the morning we went shopping in Tence and managed to buy fresh bread for the first time since leaving the South of France, and some butter and cheese as well. While we were wandering through the streets the Foreign Legion drove by in convoy and spotted us amongst the cheering crowds all shouting: '*Vive Spears*' which gave us a great moral uplift. After our successful shopping we joined the Spearhead convoy for a drive of about 120 kilometres which took us through St Etienne, the black country of France: coal mines, factories and chimneys belching soot and smoke. It was pouring with rain but that did not deter the crowds of people lining the streets waving flags and cheering. Whenever we slowed down, fruit, cakes and messages of good luck written on postcards were thrown into our car; when we stopped completely we were offered a variety of alcoholic drinks. No wonder the convoy became more and more ragged as the number of stops increased!

13

LYONS

Our flying column was heading with all speed towards L'Arbresèle, some 15 kilometres from Lyons. Lyons was still in the hands of the Germans, and we had orders to capture it before they could blow up all the bridges over the rivers Saône and Rhône.

We installed the hospital in a largish hotel which, although full of residents, was the only possible building. The proprietor and his wife were most co-operative and let us have the dining room which we divided into a ward and operating theatre. We removed all the furniture and hung curtains to separate the theatre from the ward. Wounded began to arrive before we had finished unpacking our equipment. Later in the afternoon two young SS officers were brought in. They were both young, blond, very good looking and very arrogant – typical Hitler, Aryan types. Both were badly wounded. One was abdominal, the other had multiple injuries. They both spoke excellent English and I told them I was going to give them transfusions of plasma before I sent them to the operating theatre. They demanded to know and be reassured that the plasma did not come from Jewish, Negro or any other 'foreign' blood. As the plasma was supplied to us by the Americans I told them where it had originated and therefore could not guarantee that it was pure Aryan. They both refused the plasma despite the fact that I told them they would probably die if they did not receive it as they had both lost a great deal of blood. Sadly, they both died. Perhaps they would have done anyway but I wondered afterwards if I should have lied to them. At the time I felt no pity as I had seen too many deaths and heard of the terrible atrocities the SS had committed in France.

We worked flat out until the early hours of the morning receiving, among other wounded, eighteen grands blessés who were all hospitalised, the remainder being evacuated to a civilian hospital some way behind the front line. The proprietor and his wife worked all night with us, helping in every way they could without hindering us. The fact that we had electricity and running water certainly helped as well.

Joan and I found a room for ourselves in a smaller hotel across the street from the hospital and crawled into bed at about 3am. It was a very comfortable bedroom with enormous pink quilts on the beds and lace curtains at the windows. It was equipped with a wash basin but, alas, no water and the only lavatory was behind the bar. It was a stinking squatter and had to be used by everyone, resident and visitor. However, we only slept there and were back at the hospital at dawn. Three more wounded had arrived during our absence and while we were gulping down some hot strong coffee another full ambulance arrived. There were two head cases who died almost immediately and a légionnaire with his arms, legs and hands shot to pieces. The Colonel started to operate on him while we were still giving him plasma. He collapsed half way through the operation; as we had no blood available the Colonel ordered us to take a pint of his own blood and transfuse it to the patient while he continued to operate. We very unwillingly did this and, the operation completed, we returned the légionnaire to the ward where, in spite of everything, he continued to haemorrhage. The Colonel ordered us to take another pint of his blood and this time Joan and I refused. He was furious with us and returned to the theatre. While Joan gave plasma to another patient, I sent the innkeeper's wife running through the village to find another universal donor. Luckily she found one quickly and we were able to save the légionnaire's life. The Colonel calmed down and admitted later that if he had collapsed we would have been without a surgeon for the other wounded. At the same time I don't think he would ever have forgiven us if the légionnaire had died.

We operated until two o'clock and then received orders to move on to Lyons, which was in the process of being liberated. All the patients were immediately evacuated to a civilian hospital at St Etienne and by four o' clock the hotel was empty. At five o'clock we were on the road heading for Lyons.

We reached the suburbs of Lyons very quickly. Only half the town had been captured. There was fierce fighting near the bridges, most of which had been blown up by the Germans in spite of the speed of the spearhead. Many of the streets had been blocked by barricades and as we continued towards the centre of the town small groups of FFI were hiding in doorways and behind sandbags letting their guns off at nothing in particular. A pontoon bridge had been hastily constructed by the Sappers and we were floated across on it.

We drove as quickly as we were able to, hoping by speed to avoid the sniping which, apart from the trigger-happy FFI, seemed to be coming from the roof tops.

We drove to the military hospital in one of the main squares where, after an inspection, the Colonel decided that they had ample staff and facilities to deal with the injured and did not need our help. Then we went in search of accommodation and ended up at the Claridges Hotel near the centre of the town. There was neither water nor electricity but with no wounded to care for our comfort was unimportant. The hotelier and his wife seemed friendly and gave us each a room. There were all sorts of rumours flying around, one being that the top floor was still occupied by Germans. Although we didn't believe this we did take the precaution of locking the doors of our rooms.

After dumping our belongings we set off in the jeep to see how the battle was progressing. Colonel de Lange, commanding the Foreign Legion, passed us in his scout car and our Colonel said brightly: 'We'll follow him. Wherever the Legion is it will be safe.' I never did figure out whether or not that was meant as a compliment to the Legion. All the same, the farther we followed de Lange the thicker the bullets flew and I was not enjoying it at all, especially as we had no cover on the jeep. As I was sitting next to Terramorsi, who was driving, I persuaded him to lose de Lange and return to the centre of Lyons. We passed légionnaires creeping up the sides of streets and more FFI entrenched behind barricades. It was amusing to watch them duck their heads every time there was a burst of gunfire and then cautiously lift them up again – only to duck down again an instant later.

We found General Brosset in the main square in front of the Mairie, sitting in his jeep surrounded by an admiring crowd. We stopped and chatted with him until an extra violent volley of fire came from the houses opposite. Several people in the crowd flung themselves to the ground and women started screaming. The Colonel decided to drive off again in the direction of the firing to show the crowd that there was nothing to panic about, or so he said! I thought, but did not dare say: 'What a damn silly way to be killed' as we were sitting targets in our jeep.

We made our way to another square where a hated 'Milice' had just been captured. The fury of the crowd was frightening and quite sickening. The Colonel insisted on watching. The man was pushed into a sack which was tied at the top with a piece of rope. He was then thrown into the middle of the crowd, like a fox to a pack of hounds. They kicked, stamped and jumped on him and every so often he was thrown into the air and came crashing on to the pavement to the accompaniment of shouts and invectives.

After this exhibition of mass hysteria we found a large bistro crammed full with a wildly excited crowd. Joan and I were snatched up in the middle of it and embraced by what seemed like hundreds of people and passed from shoulder to shoulder while everyone sang the '*Marseillaise*', '*God Save the King*' and the Resistance song. It was difficult to get away but we returned to our hotel where I found a bottle of champagne hidden in my bedroom cupboard and we drank to victory.

5 September – The shooting over, Joan and I went shopping and returned with all sorts of make-up, scent, face powder, lipstick and some much needed clean underpants. A victory parade and review by General de Lattre and General Brosset was arranged for the afternoon.

At midday we assembled in Terramorsi's jeep and waited for three hours in a side street before finally receiving the order to move off in the parade we drove through the streets lined with cheering spectators. Many of them were in tears; they caught hold of our hands and arms as we slowly moved forward. Several times I was nearly pulled out of the jeep. As Joan and I were the only women in the parade we seemed to be a special target. I was so busy clinging on that I missed saluting the Generals – in fact I never saw them! By the time the parade was over we were very bruised and had fixed grins on our faces. Back at the hotel we were treated to a dinner of *pâté de foie gras* and other good things, washed down with champagne and brandy, and sang songs until midnight.

Joan and I were thanked by the Commandos and Generals Brosset and de Lattre. It had been a great adventure; we felt very privileged and hoped we had justified ourselves after the arguments I had won with the Generals who tried to prevent us from taking part in the landings in the South of France.

The next morning the Colonel sent me off in his car with the hotelier and his wife to collect his sister and her husband who lived on their farm a few kilometres outside Lyon.

Their little boy and only child had been shot and killed by the Germans two days before as he was walking through a field of corn, carrying a bottle of milk to a sick neighbour. The funeral had been arranged for that afternoon. The farmer killed a goose for us and filled the car with butter, eggs and fruit; on the return journey through one of the streets of Lyons there was a sudden burst of gunfire and my poor passengers became hysterical, shouting at me to drive faster. Having experienced the greater danger of FFI bullets and their crazily driven cars, I knew the best way was to slow down so that they could recognise the Free French car. I played the dumb *Anglaise* and pulled to a halt, waiting for the cars and bullets to whizz by and for my passengers to calm down.

Père Boileau arrived the following morning and told us where the hospital was encamped. On the seventh, Biddy and Jean arrived to collect Joan and me; we all got a very cool reception for creeping away in the middle of the night to join the Commandos.

On the eve of our return to the hospital the Colonel set off with two cars to try and collect replacements for Thibaux, Coupigny and Guyon who had all asked to be transferred due to the Colonel's trip to the Commandos.

He was pressed for time and could not risk a breakdown, so I drove him in his requisitioned car and Iris and Kit followed in La Belle Marguerite. We left at five o'clock and after driving flat out for about three hours we pulled to the side of the road to refuel and have a bite to eat. As soon as we set off again there was a clatter and bang and Marguerite came to an abrupt halt in the middle of the road. Her track rod had broken and her front wheels had done the splits. Kit and Iris would certainly have been killed if this had happened when they were doing 80 miles an hour.

We left them to extricate themselves and continued on our way. We reached Aix at two in the morning and the Colonel persuaded one of his friends to come to his aid. After the necessary papers were signed we drove on through the night to Marseilles and another friend of the Colonel's where we spent the remainder of the night. He was less successful here but signed up another surgeon from the hospital at Marseilles in the morning and we were back at the unit by late afternoon.

9 September – The hospital was all under tents, except for the female personnel. We were lodged in great comfort in single rooms in the château which was inhabited by a very kind old Comtesse. She gave us the use of her dining room for the officers' mess and we were waited upon by an immaculate butler wearing white gloves and livery – serving bully beef and army rations! The Comtesse seemed very old to us; she had witnessed both World Wars and regaled us with stories of the first.

I was really pleased not to be living out of a haversack and to be back with old friends again. I spent most of this, my first full day back, sorting out my clothes and washing the filthy ones I had worn for nearly a month, and reading a pile of letters which had accumulated during my absence.

10 September – Our petrol arrived and we moved at once to a small village called Buxy, the other side of Macon. We installed ourselves in the empty, dilapidated Château de Crey where the five drivers – Biddy, Iris, Kit, Rosie and me – were huddled together at the top of the house in one bare, leaky room.

The Château de Crey was surrounded by parkland and green meadows. In the evening, I went for a walk through the fields and filled my cap with mushrooms. A kind peasant woman gave me two eggs so that I was able to make a mushroom omelette for the five of us – a pleasant change from army rations.

An Englishwoman turned up at the hospital in the morning. She had heard there were some English women at the hospital and we were the first she had met since the Germans had invaded France. She was married to a Frenchman and had been in the Resistance and captured by the Gestapo. She showed us her hands. Her finger nails had been pulled out one by one as they tortured her. The nails showed no sign of growing again. She told us some horrifying stories of German atrocities. We gave her some army rations. She had no idea whether her husband, who had also been in the Resistance, was alive or dead.

11 September – As we were still short of petrol the Colonel sent a forward unit, consisting of 22 personnel, to accompany the Deuxième Dragoons who were due to go into action that night. The Deuxième Dragoons was a unit formed entirely of escapees from occupied France to North Africa who escaped to join the Free French. Their orders were to cover the left of the Second Army Corps where thousands of Germans were trying to escape north.

12 September – On the road again through Beaune, Nuits St George and Clos Vougeot, famous names of Burgundy wines. Our destination was Montmuzzard, the military hospital situated at the farther side of Dijon. We arrived before the division and nearly caught up with the retreating Germans.

The hospital was vast and had been evacuated by the Germans only a few hours before we arrived. The Colonel had to get rid of a curious collection of humanity who had taken up residence in the comparative safety of a hospital – tramps, thieves, collaborators and civilian personnel who were employed by the Germans in running the hospital, Franc Tireurs, partisans, all of different creeds and politics and all fighting among themselves. There were also nuns, priests, *service sanitaire*, *etc*. The Colonel turned them all out except the few who had always worked in the hospital. There were a number of German wounded who had been left behind and nine corpses. I had to drive Duprez round Dijon so that he could arrange for their disposal.

13 September – I drove Duprez and the Mayor of Dijon to look for a petrol dump which was reputed to be hidden near an aerodrome. We drove through Beaune and followed a canal to Auton. We found and searched two aerodromes but found no trace of any petrol. I must admit that I was half-hearted during the search. I kept thinking of the poor boys of Le Lavandou and didn't want the same fate.

On our way back we stopped at a small inn where we had a delicious meal of home made pâté, ham and mirabelle tart. When we had finished, the innkeeper's wife gave us a present of eggs, butter and milk for the hospital.

As we were leaving, a girl on a bicycle came rushing up to us saying she had just passed a number of Germans coming up the road towards us. Duprez got his revolver out and I drove slowly up the road. We saw nothing except signs of recent fighting, dead horses and dead Germans. We heard a shot which seemed to come from behind a hedge and immediately afterwards I had a flat back tyre. I drove quite a long way before stopping! When I changed the wheel I found a long-nosed bullet in it.

From midday on the twelfth the hospital had been filling up with patients. The numbers increased daily until we had a total of 266 admissions, of whom 200 had been wounded in battle. Their nationalities showed the diverse complexities of the liberation of Burgundy and of the 'mopping up' of the surrounding countryside and forests. 160 of the wounded came from our division, and 60 from the German Army and included Germans, Austrians, Czechs, Poles and Russians. 40 were Resistance fighters and one an American parachutist. Several of the wounded were exhausted, having had to walk long distances to the hospital because the shortage of petrol had grounded the divisional ambulances.

The town of Dijon was the scene of the misfortunes of the German occupation and the hospital reflected some of these. For example, we were obliged to have armed guards in the wards to protect our patients from marauding bands of so-called Resistance fighters who were ready to take revenge on anyone. We also had to have armed guards patrolling the outside of the hospital to prevent pilfering and the dumping of corpses into a stock of coffins which had been left behind by the Germans. Isolated wounded Germans, dressed in civilian clothes, were frequently deposited at the hospital or came by themselves seeking protection. I was again working half the time at the hospital and half undertaking driving duties.

The following afternoon I drove the Colonel, Iris and Edith to the square outside the Préfecture of Dijon where a stage and seats had been erected. We had been invited, together with the entire population of Dijon to witness the ceremony of head shaving, tarring and feathering of the female collaborators of the city. I found it quite repellent and returned to the car after watching the first few of these wretched women who, with their hands tied behind their backs, were made to kneel down in the midst of the jeering crowd. Their heads were then shaved except for a top-knot, after which they were tarred and feathered. The obvious enjoyment of the crowd was the most sickening part of it. The male collaborators were simply taken out and shot. At least we were spared from seeing this.

16 September – General Ralenger paid us a visit in the evening and told us the latest battle plans for the division and how the attack was being delayed through lack of petrol and munitions. He also told us that all the black troops in the division were to be returned to their home lands of the Cameroons and Chad, as it was feared they would be unable to withstand the rigours of a European winter. This meant we would lose our 69 Tirailleurs who had been with us all the way

through the Western desert and the Italian campaigns and who had worked uncomplainingly in the kitchens, the mess, the hospital wards and the laundry. Most of all we would miss our particular orderlies and friends Jean and Michel who kept our tents clean and tidy and looked after us as if we were their own family.

17 September – I had the day off and decided to do a little reconnoitring on my own. I went to Nuits St George where I persuaded the wine merchants to give me several cases of red and white wine for the hospital and a case of champagne for ourselves, which made me very popular while it lasted.

The countryside around Dijon was completely different from the South of France up to Lyons. We really did not have much time to do any sightseeing or take in the landscape or anything else until we reached Burgundy. Here the land was divided into what appeared to be small plots, never more than a few acres of vines, each bearing the name of a famous Burgundy wine. It was a very rich part of France and a gourmet's paradise, as we were soon to discover.

Our petrol arrived at last; we handed over to 405 Base Hospital and left at midday. I drove the Colonel and Frankau ahead of the convoy to the small village of Villersexel, 30 kilometres from Belfort. We found a huge château, ideal for the entire hospital. The Colonel left Frankau on guard in case some other unit claimed it, while I drove him back to the convoy and we all arrived in very good order by 7pm.

The Château de Gramont at Villersexel belonged to one of the oldest and grandest families in France and was historically famous as well. The Comtesse de Gramont and her daughter-in-law were living in the chateau. They turned out to be the least co-operative and most inhospitable of all the people we came in contact with in France.

The château was a perfect place for a hospital. Its wide drives and large courtyard provided plenty of space for the ambulances to park and turn round. The château itself was large enough for all our needs; the wards were all on the first floor in small bedrooms and the operating theatre in a minute study on the ground floor next to an enormous dining room, which we were permitted to use only as our mess. A huge dining table, and equally large serving tables, overlooked by the portraits of generations of Gramonts, made our tin plates and mugs look slightly out of place.

The X-ray equipment was installed amid piled-up furniture in one of the annexes and the pharmacy was equally badly housed in a beautiful library where there was very little space. The Comtesse would not allow us room for more than 100 beds in her château and so, in spite of the rain and cold, two large tents were put up in the park for the medical and lightly wounded cases. They were heated by paraffin stoves kept going full blast day and night; even so, we could not keep out the damp and cold, or the mud. We women were housed in the servants' rooms on the top floor: small mean rooms, devoid of furniture and bitterly cold, without water, heating or light until our own hospital generator and wiring was connected.

The reception and resuscitation wards were squashed together in an alcove under the splendid staircase of honour. We only had room for two trestles for the transfusion stretchers and about six stretchers on the ground, packed together like sardines. As usual I worked in the resuscitation ward with Joan – eight hours on and eight hours off.

Once the rush of wounded began, it was absolute chaos, with the stretchers two deep along the entrance passage where they had to wait their turn for treatment, with nurses, orderlies and doctors falling over them and each other. Getting the stretchers up the grand staircase was difficult too as the stairs were very steep and full of sharp corners.

We never understood why the Colonel suffered the Comtesse as he did. He had the authority to requisition whatever he required and he could have turned her out of her grand château if he had wanted to. Instead he put up with her outrageous behaviour, even going so far as to send her to Paris in one of our staff cars (driven, I think, by Rosie) on the understanding that we could use the dining room as another ward. On her return from Paris she informed him that she had changed her mind and he could not have it after all, which he accepted. We came to the conclusion that he must have had a reason that we knew nothing about, or was intimidated by her rank and riches.

The Comtesse and her daughter-in-law never came near the hospital, never visited the wounded, never offered to help in any way whatsoever. They were aggressively anti-British and frequently accused us of stealing their fruit and flowers. They even accused us of stealing their wood when we collected fallen branches off the ground for kindling. What they never discovered was that, as it became progressively colder, one of the woodmen took pity on us and used to leave a pile of logs hidden in one of the outhouses for us to collect. The Comtesse and her daughter-in-law were, fortunately, the exception to the rule but sadly many of the French aristocracy behaved badly during the occupation.

Thanks to the friendly woodman, we were able to have fires in our bedroom grates, which kept us from freezing and enabled us to dry our often soaking wet uniforms.

The shortage of petrol continued and during this period we only had enough for one staff car to be used daily.

The same day that we arrived at Villersexel the forward unit, which had been stationed in Montbozen, was moved forward again to the civilian hospital at Lure which had been liberated the same day. The forward unit was increased in size, with the addition of Evelyn and Edith as sisters, Kit as driver and Thibaux as head surgeon, with several more orderlies.

The division was so severely hampered by lack of petrol that they could only send out patrols to harass the Germans. Because of this, they suffered heavy casualties. Their objective was to take Belfort and to close the Belfort Gap, which was strongly defended by seven German divisions, well dug in, with heavily fortified gun emplacements surrounded by mine fields.

Between 19 and 27 September I worked entirely in the resuscitation ward in conditions almost as hectic as at Le Lavandou, not through lack of personnel so much as lack of space. With the overcrowding in the passages it was difficult to spot the urgent cases and we were continually falling over one another. It was almost impossible to keep our annexe warm, even with the two paraffin stoves; there were so many draughty passages and doors leading out of it.

One morning a légionnaire was brought in with a flesh wound in his arm and a suspected fracture of his collar bone. He was moaning and groaning to such an extent that I asked the Colonel to examine him in case his injuries were more serious than they seemed. The Colonel said his collar bone was not broken; all he needed was a couple of stitches in his arm and he could return to his unit. The soldier continued to moan and groan; the Colonel said to him: 'Pull yourself together, you're making more fuss than an Italian.' The soldier replied: 'Please sir, I *am* an Italian.'

The weather became increasingly cold and wet. Very soon the staff cars and trucks became bogged down in the mud and we had difficulty in starting them in the mornings. The beautiful courtyard was churned up by the endless convoys of ambulances.

Biddy and I found a small village shop where we were able to buy butter and cheese from an old Frenchman. He was very proud of having taught himself English from a library of Shakespeare's plays. We were the first English he had met and he was delighted to try to converse with us. Unfortunately, Shakespearean English pronounced in French was completely incomprehensible and neither of us could understand a word he said. He made it very clear that he considered us both idiots and that the fault was ours.

During the time I was working in reception René was brought in with seven broken ribs and innumerable bruises. His driver had been shot and killed beside him and his jeep overturned in a ditch. The Colonel strapped him up and admitted him to Betty's ward, but he insisted on discharging himself the next day.

By this time all our Tirailleurs had departed and been replaced by an odd assortment of untrained enthusiasts and fifteen German and

Austrian prisoners of war. They were all lightly wounded cases who had been admitted to the hospital and were never officially declared cured. They remained with us until the end of the war. They were fitted out in American uniforms and worked for us as stretcher bearers, cleaners and grave diggers. To begin with they were guarded, because of the proximity of the German lines, but it soon became clear that they had no intention of escaping to fight again and the guards were withdrawn.

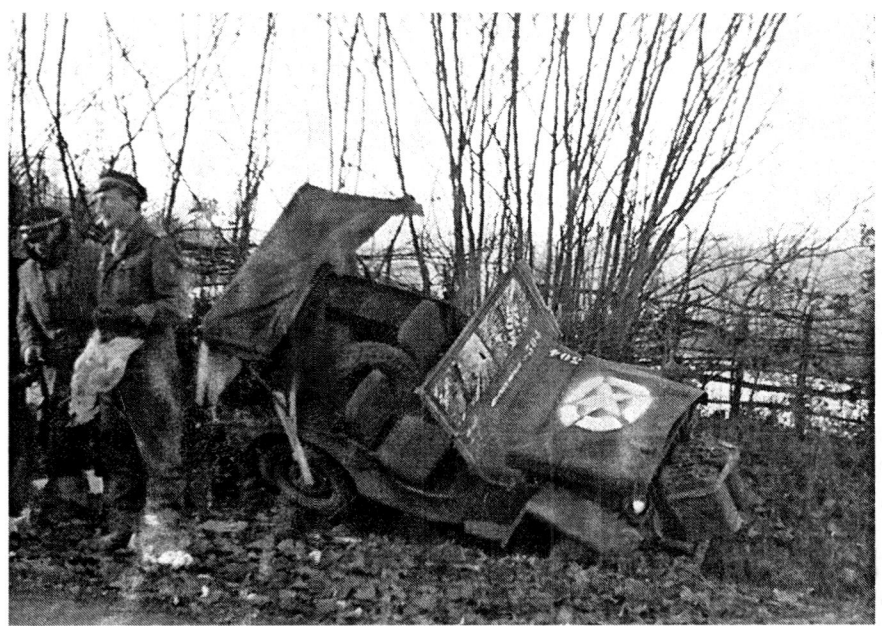

René's jeep blown up by a land mine.

14

Home Leave

The hospital settled down again to its familiar routine. The division could not go into action for lack of petrol but patrols were sent out daily and both the hospitals became busy. The objective of the division was Belfort and the Belfort Gap, into Alsace, which was heavily defended by seven divisions of Germans distributed in the surrounding forest with gun emplacements, mines and forts. The Colonel seemed to be ill and tired after all the stress and worry from the officers and staff caused by the Commando jaunt. He lost two stone in weight and his cheery character. Thibaux returned and carried out most of the operations. It became bitterly cold and everyone seemed to be suffering from colds and coughs including me.

I had been alternating from working in the hospital and driving and did the post several times, much to the indignation of Jocelyn who looked upon it as her perk. She enjoyed chatting up all the officers at HQ, most of all St Hilier, who she had set her cap at. He had a perfectly good wife and children and I didn't think he would leave them for her. Biddy and I shared a room at the top of the chateau. Thank goodness, she had at last forgiven me for going off with the Commandos without telling her and accepted firstly that I was forbidden to tell anyone, and secondly that she was away on leave when I left. Our room was cold and airless but, with the help of the head woodsman, we were able to light a fire at night. I found a sick horse in a field but was unable to find its owner and it eventually died. The French didn't seem to care much about their animals when they were sick, and left them to die.

6 October – General de Lattre inspected the hospital and decorated several of the wounded. He had lunch with us afterwards so we had to wear our best uniforms and stand in line to be inspected – something we hated doing.

7 October – Iris and Mergier turned up just as Biddy was setting off to look for them. They had reached Paris without too much trouble. They had dumped the old Comtesse at her house near the Rue de Varenne, and Mergier with his parents, who put Kit and Iris up for the night. On their return journey Marguerite broke down but they managed to get her going again after some time. They were then run

into by a truck which buckled the car's mudguard and bonnet. They managed to get a tow to a garage where they left Kit to supervise the repairs. We opened a bottle of champagne to celebrate their return.

10 October – The Colonel sent Biddy and me to collect his parents from Chambon in his own car and drive them back to their house near Marseilles. We left at 7am and drove 400 kilometres, arriving at their house in the afternoon. We spent the night with them and, although we were up early next morning, it took until 11 o'clock to pack everything into and on the car. Monsieur Vernier was very old and pale and confused. His wife seemed to be younger and took care of her husband, organised everything and encouraged us all. She had been up all night getting their belongings packed and her schoolmaster son had filled every available space in the car with packages. He had even tied bundles on to the mudguards and two mattresses on to the roof. The car looked more like a gypsy caravan than a military staff car. Somehow we managed to 'shoe-horn' the old couple into the back of the car among squawking chickens, baskets, bags and suitcases. In the front of the car we had cans of petrol jammed between our legs and more of their packages stacked around us.

The first half of the journey was along narrow twisty mountainous roads and with our overloaded car we were obliged to travel very slowly. We frequently had to stop for the old man to get out to have a pee. Each time it took ages to disentangle him and then repack him again. We also wasted nearly an hour eating an enormous picnic lunch Madame Vernier had prepared for us.

Once in the Rhône valley, along straighter roads, our speed increased but we were held up a long time at Avignon waiting to cross the river by the only ferry. We had four hours driving with very poor lights before we finally arrived at their house at midnight. I fell asleep immediately in their spare room.

Next morning we were up at seven o'clock to find Madame Vernier already up and cooking a breakfast of porridge and coffee while we unloaded the car and carried all the belongings into their house. We were able to get away by nine and made the journey back to the hospital in twelve hours, much to the surprise of the Colonel who had not expected to see us for another day. The lights of the car had failed completely in the end and we had to drive by the light of a torch hung out of the window. Apart from this problem the Colonel's car went like a bird.

Upon our return we found there were three different rows going on. 1 – The colonel was trying to change the hospital into a *Corp de L'Armée* hospital. 2 – David Siggs had taken my 82, without permission, to drive Duprez somewhere. I joined in the row as I was responsible for 82 and no one, and I repeated no one, other than us drivers was allowed to drive our cars. It only happened because Kit, Biddy and I were away and Iris was out at the time. 3 — Jean was furious because Françoise, who had no nursing training, had been put in reception without her knowledge. As Jean was Head Sister and responsible for all appointments she had every reason to be furious.

11 October — The Colonel sent a second forward unit to Luxeuil-les-Bains. It was housed in the Château de Brouches which was owned and inhabited by a very old lady who was extremely dignified and patriotic. She enjoyed comparing the three German–Franco wars she had lived though and I visited her whenever I could to listen to her stories, which I found fascinating. Thibaux was put in charge of the second unit and started operating three days later.

The hospital was now split into three sections: 100 beds and personnel, at the main hospital at Villersexel, 40 beds and personnel at Lure and 30 beds and personnel at Brouches — 170 beds in all. We admitted 650 wounded and a few medical cases as well.

The German army, against which our division was fighting, included several regiments of the dreaded SS who succeeded in infiltrating our lines. No one knew where they would turn up next. Because of them we were ordered to wear our tin hats whenever we were driving our cars. I took my revolver as well!

Jocelyn returned one morning very cross. She had bullet holes in her beloved 64 but neither was any the worse. She said when she heard the first shot she put her foot down on the accelerator and sped off down the road.

The division was still hampered by a lack of petrol and munitions, which had to be ferried up from the Mediterranean. During this campaign we suffered the highest death rate of the war. Out of the 1,650 wounded we admitted in our three units, 81 died and the deaths on the battlefield were more than double this number.

Meanwhile the battle for Belfort swayed backwards and forwards. One day the division would advance three miles and the next it would be pushed back four. It was during this advancing and retreating that I came the nearest to being taken prisoner. We had a small boy in the hospital who had been wounded in the head by a shell splinter during a skirmish around the village where he lived. When we received orders to move up to join our number two forward unit at Lure all the patients had to be evacuated. I was told to return the boy to his family as he was well on the road to recovery. He lived at Faymont, which was about ten kilometres from Villersexel. As it was very near the front line I checked with HQ to be certain that I could get through. They told me it was now well behind our lines and there was no danger of running into Germans – apart from the odd SS. I made a slight detour round one village as there seemed to be a certain amount of gunfire in the vicinity and stopped at the next to ask a local how much further away the village was. He said that it was only about another mile but that it had been re-taken by the Germans. I did not believe him and continued on my way. Not long afterwards I met a group of infantrymen who told me that it was quite safe to continue to Faymont as it had been re-taken by our troops that morning.

As I approached the village the countryside suddenly became ominously silent, in the way battle areas are; no animals in the fields, no men working, no smoke from the chimneys and no children playing in front of houses – in fact, no sign of life at all. I came to an army barricade across the road and asked the sergeant how much farther down the road Faymont was. He told me about 500 metres and lifted the barrier for me to pass. Round the next bend I passed a gun emplacement whose crew looked at me rather curiously but said nothing. I drove round a blind corner and came face to face with a platoon of Germans marching towards me. I jammed the car into reverse and shot backwards round the bend as fast as the car would go and did not stop until I reached the gun emplacement. The Germans must have been as surprised to see me as I was to see them as they did not open fire. I told the gunners what I had seen and they said they were a bit surprised to see me drive past and thought I must be driving a General on inspection. Back at the road block they asked to see my *ordre de mission*, which struck me as a bit ironical.

Studying my map again I found another road to Faymont and started down it. This time I was brought to an abrupt halt at another road block and no argument would persuade the Sergeant to let me through without a pass from HQ. Back at the Command post I asked them to show me on my map exactly where the front line was and whether Faymont was in our hands or not. I was shown the latest movement map and they told me that Faymont had been re-taken by the Germans an hour before I had driven down the road.

I managed to find some people in the last village I had driven through before the barrier who knew the boy and his parents. They promised to look after him and to contact his family at once, so I left him with them.

Arriving back at the hospital during lunch I told the Colonel, rather crossly, about my narrow squeak. I also felt guilty about failing in my mission and having to dump the boy on neighbours. The Colonel only laughed at me and said I was 'chicken', which wasn't very nice of him. Later in the day he apologised and said that the village had indeed fallen to the enemy and that the Germans had advanced six miles before being pushed back again.

29 October – A month's home leave was being offered to all of us in turn on condition that we found our own way to England and back again. Edith, Kelsey and I accepted the first trip. In great excitement I got 82 ready for the journey to Paris and packed my bag.

30 October – We left early in the morning and arrived in Paris at three o'clock – my first visit. We had a very smooth drive, except that a black hen flew into the windscreen and cracked it. Edith, who was sitting in the front beside me, immediately announced that it was the worst possible omen and that something terrible would happen to us all. I tersely told her that it was her side of the windscreen and nothing to do with Kelsey or me but secretly I agreed with her and felt very spooky.

I contacted Rosie who was in Paris waiting for our arrival so that she could return to the hospital in 82. She had earlier skidded her car (72) off the road on her way to Paris and it was doubtful it could be repaired. Pierre Mergier's parents generously put us all up in their comfortable flat in Neuilly.

31 October – I spent most of the day visiting endless French bureaux trying to get passages for the three of us.

I collected the car and left the Nannies with the Mergiers. After calling for Rosie from her aunt's palatial house in the Rue de Varenne, we went off to the French Air Ministry. After a long wait there, and at the American and RAF HQs, we finally got passages on a British Army flight leaving the following day.

1 November – We finally boarded an old British army plane leaving for England at 1.30. Rosie drove us to the army airfield, two hours from Paris. We climbed into an old DC3 full of soldiers and kit bags, most of whom got off the plane at Cherbourg. We continued to a military airfield somewhere in England. We landed in the dark and, after signing our names and handing over our mail for posting, were driven by bus to Audley Street and dumped on the pavement. Edith and Kelsey seemed to be completely lost, so I found a taxi and took them with me to the Berkeley Hotel, changed some francs into pounds sterling, lent them enough for their accommodation for the night and waved them goodbye. I hoped that my responsibilities for them were over until the return journey. I was thankful that the black hen, which none of us had forgotten, had not prevented us from arriving in England.

I wasted precious hours of my leave arranging for our passage back which was eventually provided for us by the RAF, the French HQ only

offering us a crossing by boat, which I refused. Apart from that, I
visited my family, met many friends, got in two days' hunting,
collected warm woollies for the hospital personnel from the Canadian
Red Cross, and experienced the first doodlebugs and V2s in London –
which I found far more terrifying than shell or mortar fire. I did not
fit into life with my parents at all – they were more interested in when
the sweep was coming or that I had eaten their ration of butter than in
hearing about my adventures.

On the eighteenth day I rose early and went to the Berkeley to change
into my uniform and collect the woollies I had left there. Edith and
Kelsey arrived at 11am; we went to Air Movements in Old Quebec
Street and had to hang about there getting weighed, *etc*. At midday a
bus took us to an aerodrome, a two-hour journey. After passing
through a security check and drinking a cup of coffee we boarded the
plane at 3pm.
    It was a much more comfortable plane than the one we had left on.
Instead of the old bucket seats of the DC3 we had proper seats with
seat belts. The flight was bumpy so we had to keep the belts on for the
entire journey. We landed at an aerodrome some two hours from Paris
and were driven to the centre of the city in an army bus.
    Rosie was waiting for us with 82. Unfortunately we had to wait in
Paris for two days while her brakes and suspension were being
repaired for us by General Motors. When we collected her they would
not take any payment and even gave me some spare parts as a parting
gift. Edith and Kelsey had left before us with David Rowlands and
party.

23 November – I collected Rosie and 82 early in the morning and
after calling at various military HQs on behalf of the division we set
off for Lure where we found the hospital still in residence. I was
delighted to be back again and felt that I had been living in an unreal
world during my leave. Only Flick understood a little of what our lives
were like in the hospital. We found the hospital in good heart and
working as hard as ever.
    Everyone in the hospital and the division was mourning the
unfortunate death of our much beloved General Brosset who had
drowned in tragic circumstances. He was driving his jeep with his
ADC, Jean-Pierre Aumont (actor and film star) seated beside him and
his devoted driver behind. They were on their way to inspect a section
of the front line. Brosset always drove like a maniac, and had written
off several jeeps and staff cars. On this particular day he got his own
jeep stuck in the mud somewhere and had promptly requisitioned
another from the Atelier Lourd but it had faulty steering. No one
could remember whether or not he had been warned about it. Near the

front line he came across a detachment of Sappers in the process of de-mining a small bridge over a stream which was swollen into a torrent by the heavy rainfall. They had succeeded in clearing the left-hand lane and had taped it. Brosset, driving very fast as usual, swung the jeep to the de-mined side of the bridge but the jeep, with its tricky steering and tyres thick with mud, skidded and jumped the bridge into the fast running water below.

The driver came to the surface first and was rescued, unconscious, by the Sappers. They then dragged Jean-Pierre Aumont, badly hurt and half drowned to the bank but were unaware that Brosset was in the jeep as well. Brosset was a very strong swimmer but he was pinned under the steering wheel and could also have been unconscious. The jeep was swept downstream by the current and by the time he was rescued he was already dead. The Colonel and Iris rushed over with cylinders of oxygen and spent two hours vainly trying to resuscitate him.

Brosset's body was brought back to the hospital and laid in the chapel of St Anne's Convent. He was buried between the graves of the Commandants Mirkin and Langlois at Villersexel on 24 November. The service was taken by Père Hirleman, Chaplain to the division. Everyone from Spears who was able to attend was there, together with as many officers and men who could be spared from the division which was in full attack, carrying out the last battle orders of Brosset.

General Garbay succeeded General Brosset in command of the division. He had a very different personality. He was extremely reserved, almost shy, and lacked his predecessor's sparkle and dynamism. We rarely saw him and had the feeling that he did not really approve of us and our unusual circus.

25 November – Terramorsi turned up at the hospital with an unexpected present which was sent, according to him, from the Vercours Maquis for me. It was a car he had had repainted in khaki with the divisional and hospital numbers on its mudguards, as well as the Free French Croix de Lorraine and the Hadfield–Spears badge. It looked very smart indeed.

I was delighted to have my own little car to run about in when I was off duty. I took Rosie and Biddy for a drive in her and she went like a bird. She was a useful addition to our war-weary staff cars and easily earned her keep. I christened her 'Buzz' and brought her back to England at the end of the war.

7 December – A day's leave. René collected me in his jeep and drove me to the front line to show me where his regiment had fought and won their bloodiest battle. We drove along the most appalling tracks while he pointed out various battles and landmarks.

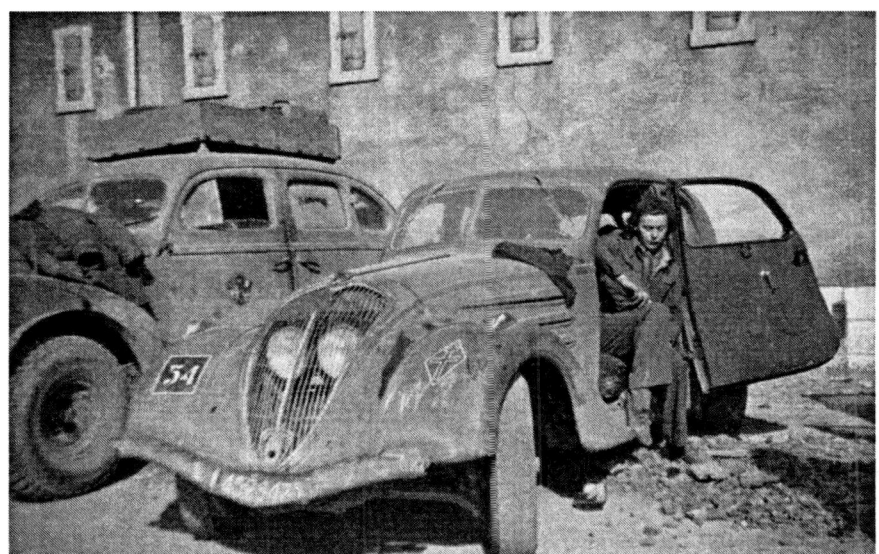

Rosie in the author's car Buzz.

At the small village of Rougemen.t we called in at a château belonging to his aunt who was still living there. She nearly fainted when she saw him and after drinking her health with some of her home-made kirsch we all went off to a small bistro for lunch. After lunch we dropped 'Tante Berthe' off at her château and made our way to another section of the front line, near Thanne, which was still in German hands.

We were given a conducted tour by a young Fusilier Marin who kept telling me to keep my head down. We saw the Germans watching us from their tanks, hull down, on the opposite hill. We walked round a captured tank which still had the charred remains of its crew on board. The Captain and René insisted that I put my feet exactly in their footsteps. I thought these instructions were to impress me until René picked up a stone and threw it a good many yards away. As it hit the ground it exploded a mine which went off with a loud bang and started the Germans firing in our direction. We crept back again with our heads well down – particularly mine. We visited the battle HQ, which was in a concrete pillbox covering a water cistern, reached by an iron ladder. By the time we had finished looking at the latest plan of attack it was dark so we left.

We had dinner with Tante Berthe. Afterwards she gave us jars of mirabelle jam and peaches and plums in brandy to take back with us. We arrived at the hospital after a scary drive, bumping into convoys and another jeep head on. I made up my mind that if I ever went for another trip with René I would do the driving.

16 December – Off to Paris after all with Mergier and Colonel Mondain in place of our Colonel. The hospital moved off at the same time, not further into Alsace but in quite another direction – somewhere near Cognac on the Atlantic coast. We stopped beyond Sens and had a really excellent meal at a café – fish, butter, eggs and lots of cream.

Had trouble-free run to Paris until we got to within 50 kilometres of the city when 82 began pulling very badly and finally pegged out on the wrong side of the Porte d'Italie. I spent an hour and a half trying to get her to go, but in vain. We managed to push her into a civilian garage for the night and continued our journey by bus and metro. Mergier took me to his parents for the night.

17 December (Saturday) – I went to General Motors, which was closed except for one mechanic who promised to keep the garage open for me and to work on the car if I could get it to him. I then went to the American Army garage where they were able to loan me a breakdown lorry and driver to tow 82 to General Motors. I got her there at midday and, with the help of the mechanic and his two friends, we took the engine to bits and put it together again. Without knowing why, we managed to get her going again. I then set off to get enough petrol coupons to get us to Cognac next day.

18 December – Left Paris with my passengers plus a French girl, Denise, who was to work in the hospital. She was one of several allotted to us since our arrival in France, much to the annoyance of Lady Spears and ourselves. We arrived at Cognac well after dark with no lights, and practically no brakes, and stayed in a small hotel.

After her service, 82 broke down on the return journey and I had to be towed back. Our poor old cars had done such an enormous mileage under every sort of condition from the sand of the desert to snow and ice in northern France that they were wearing out in spite of our care and replacement parts. In fact, about the only original bits of them were their chassis. In the afternoon I collected my things and went to the annexe again.

19 December – Set off early and called in on General Ralinger and General de Larminat to find out the whereabouts of the hospital. We reached it soon afterwards; it was installed in a civilian hospital at Saintes. General de Larminat briefed us on the reason for our sudden switch from one side of France to the other, galloping off in what appeared to be the opposite direction to the battle zone. He explained that a strong pocket of Germans was ensconced at Royan Pointe de Grave and, although they were completely encircled, they were resisting with force, protected by a concrete fortification and deep

minefields, and benefiting from the natural defence of islands and swamps.

Their position enabled them to prevent the Allies from using the Atlantic ports from La Rochelle to Bordeaux – one of the reasons for our lack of petrol. Units of the Resistance under the command of General de Larminat had no modern equipment to do more than contain the Germans, therefore our Divisions had been transferred to complete the mopping up.

The *Maison de Retraite* hospital, which had been assigned to Spears, had been occupied by Germans, French Tireurs, Partisans and the FFI and was in a filthy condition and occupied mainly by patients suffering from skin and venereal diseases. It was inadequately staffed by the local Red Cross, who had little idea of hygiene or discipline. Patients came and went as they pleased. In one ward there was even a goat tied to the end of the bed of a peasant, assuring him of his ration of milk. Everyone in Spears turned to and helped clean and disinfect the wards and the majority of the FFI patients were discharged.

As the hospital's VD medical officer, Solly Albert was put in charge of the Annexe for the VD patients at La Chapelle des Pots, some 5 kilometres away from Saintes. I was sent there as his driver.

The Annexe, which had been a sanatorium in peace time, was situated in the middle of a large wood in beautiful surroundings but it was bitterly cold inside with no heating or hot water and everything was in a fine muddle. An old matron was in charge of six Red Cross nurses who were full of good will but had little experience of nursing and knew nothing about antiseptics. I was the only Spearette there and thankful to be back at my official job of driving and having nothing to do with the wards.

I had a nice bedroom to myself and, with my camp bed, orange boxes for furniture and my Tunisian fibre mats on the floor, was very comfortable. I took 82 with me and left Buzz in the care of Iris.

23 December – I took the old matron to the hospital at Sainte in the morning to collect stores and medical supplies for the Annexe. In the afternoon she accompanied me to Cognac where we called on Madame Hennessy who lived in a large château overlooking the town. The Hennessy family did not appear to have suffered greatly from the occupation. Liveried menservants opened the front door to us and we were conducted into an impressive drawing room full of priceless furniture and pictures. Madame Hennessy, lying on a chaise longue, was the personification of elegance. She was very gracious to me and I obtained from her what I had gone there for – an order to collect from her usine two bottles of cognac free of charge. I invited her back to the hospital for tea and she arrived laden with cakes and more bottles of cognac and champagne.

René arrived with an enormous bottle of Vol de Nuit scent, from Guerlain, and two lipsticks for me. We dined at a small bistro and ate oysters and steak, and drank wine and cognac.

The hospital was full of rumours of an imminent move, including one that we and the division were being transferred to Belgium.

The news from the battle front was grim. Von Runstead's attack in the Ardennes had sent the Americans reeling backwards and General Patton had decided to abandon Strasbourg and the Colmar pocket. General de Gaulle energetically opposed his plan, fearful for the lives of all the Alsatians who had welcomed the Free French and knowing that harsh reprisals would be taken against them by the Germans. He claimed that a retreat would have deep moral consequences on French public opinion as well as on their armies and, most important of all, General Leclerc's division, which was holding the line south of Strasbourg, would almost certainly be taken prisoner as it would be completely surrounded if Colmar and Strasbourg were abandoned. Therefore, in spite of General Eisenhower's refusal to supply or equip both Free French divisions, we were ordered back to Alsace with all possible speed.

25 December – After celebrating midnight mass, which was followed by an enormous supper of *pâté de foie gras*, oysters, roast goose, *etc etc* with Solly and his Red Cross helpers I was ordered back to the main hospital.

Kit and I worked all Christmas day on the staff cars in an effort to have them roadworthy for the long journey in front of us. We enjoyed another Christmas feast in the evening, this time in the English tradition of roast turkey and plum pudding, with General and Madame de Larminat as our guests.

26 December – Another day's work on the cars. I took 82 to the Atelier Lourd and wangled a new battery for her and two new tyres for Buzz, who badly needed them. We packed up the cars for an early start next morning and went to bed early.

The Annexe was returned to the Red Cross. Half of the main hospital was to remain at Sainte to continue to serve General de Larminat and his FFI while the other half rushed back to Alsace with the division. For the first and only time the hospital was split in two halves, separated by 800 kilometres and serving two different armies.

27 December – We left Sainte in the freezing cold. Thibaux drove Buzz for me, and he and all the staff cars set off ahead of the convoy. We stopped at a café during the morning for a cup of coffee to warm us up and at lunchtime for a hot meal in a restaurant, which was a great improvement on cold army rations. We reached Ahan in the

Creuse in the evening and were lodged in an empty school where the two women caretakers showed us much kindness, lighting fires and preparing a hot breakfast the next morning.

28 December – Rosie was unable to get her car to start because of frozen water in the petrol system, and several of the trucks suffered from the same complaint. Because of the breakdowns our convoy left at odd hours in a very straggly procession, spending the night at Monthelon where Duprez had a hot meal waiting for us and billets in a small hotel. The stragglers turned up at intervals and by midnight everyone was accounted for.

29 December – Off at 8am with everyone moving in one convoy. We reached Dijon by 11am, where we sat and waited for further orders. We bought some cream buns and scones from a nearby pâtisserie and ate them while we waited. Our orders arrived and we left immediately for Bourbon les Bains, arriving late in the afternoon. Duprez set off to find billets for us all and I waited in my car in the main square, opposite the Mairie. The town was full of American troops, black and white, who seemed to spend their time getting drunk and fighting among themselves instead of against the Germans. Their lack of discipline and endless brawls did not endear them to the French.

While I was waiting peacefully in my car reading a book, a drunken American sergeant reeled over and started shouting obscenities at me, so I wound up my window. This infuriated him and he began banging on the door, yelling that if the door wasn't locked he would give me a lesson I would remember all my life. I told him that the door was not locked and that I had wound up my window as I did not wish to listen to his insults. He shouted that the Americans had liberated France and that they would liberate England as well. Luckily for me two US military policemen arrived at that moment and the sergeant lurched off. The mayor's wife, who had been watching the scene from her window, came out and asked if I would like to stay with her and her husband while we were at Bourbon les Bains. I accepted gratefully and told Duprez that he need not bother about a billet for me. I was given a delicious meal, had a hot bath, and tumbled into a feather bed with clean sheets.

30 December – A day's rest. I got up early to drive the Colonel to Belfort. On my way to collect 82 I came across Kit in Marguerite being towed down the main street by two horses. Even with this powerful help Marguerite refused to start. I arranged to give her a tow with 82, and then discovered that 82 would not start either. I was able to persuade the driver of an American truck to give me a tow, which did the trick for me but I had no time to help Kit as I was already late

for the Colonel. We got to Belfort for lunch with General Gerliac in his mess. We took coffee and liqueurs in his flat and then returned to Bourbon les Bains.

Upon returning to my billet in the evening I found René waiting outside. The mayor invited him in for a drink, but not to the special dinner his wife was preparing for Kit and me.

I had a bath and washed my hair in preparation for the feast, which turned out to be memorable and a miracle of French wartime ingenuity: Potage de Maison, rabbit cooked in a delicious sauce and mirabelle tart and *framboise*, that most delicate of *eaux-de-vie*. The mayor brought up from his cellar an old green bottle covered in cobwebs which, he assured me, was genuine Napoleon brandy which he was keeping to celebrate the end of the war.

31 December – The mayoress cooked me an English breakfast of porridge (goodness knows where she got it from) and fried eggs. When I thanked her and asked her why she was so kind to me, a complete stranger, she replied: 'My dear, if my daughter was in England under the same conditions, would not your mother do the same for her?' I wondered!

We left Bourbon les Bains in convoy and drove to Damas-aux-Bois where we stopped with the rest of the division. Damas was a typical Lorraine village with one main street of houses, each one with a pile of cow manure heaped up in front of the door. Jocelyn had arrived before us with Duprez and our billets were organised. Iris, Margaret and I were lodged with an old lady and we each had a bedroom to ourselves. I was the lucky one, with a fire in my room. It was the coldest day we had yet experienced, really bitter, and the only lavatory was an outside privy at the bottom of the garden, a long walk from the house. Water had to be carried in pails from the village pump, so we didn't do much washing.

Our bedrooms were above a cow byre with a trapdoor leading from each bedroom down to the cattle, whose sweet smell and warm breath wafted through the floorboards and helped to keep us warm. Our beds had soft feather mattresses which we sank into and feather eiderdowns on top, which kept out the cold very successfully. I don't think many of us saw the New Year in – I certainly didn't.

1 January 1945 – If anything, even colder. Our orders were to remain here for two or three days. There was no driving for me so I cleaned out 82's entire petrol system, endeavouring to remove all the water from her pipes.

2 January – Drove the Colonel to the HQ at Baccarat. The petrol froze in all the cars except 82 and when I returned we all tried to unfreeze

the others with hot compresses and hot water bottles. It was hard work – as soon as we unfroze one bit another froze up again.

We learned that the divisional attack ordered had had to be cancelled as half the tanks and half the tracks were frozen solid.

4 January – Moved off in convoy, except for Kit and Rosie who could not get their cars unfrozen. I led the hospital convoy and all went well until I was ordered to halt halfway up a hill to wait for the laggards of the convoy to catch up. Needless to say I got stuck in the deep snow and had to be pushed by one jeep and pulled by another to the top of the hill. The day's itinerary took us through many Alsatian towns and villages to Hohwald, our final destination.

15

ALSACE

Hohwald was a picture postcard Alsatian village, deep in snow when we arrived. Along a narrow track through woods, and a mile or so from the village, was the Convent of St Odile, the patron saint of Alsace and in peacetime a place of pilgrimage and a major tourist attraction.

The hospital was installed in the Grand Hotel in the main street; the drivers and sisters were all billeted in the Auberge Eboué. The proprietor, M Eboué, and his wife took over all the cooking for the officers' mess which was in the dining room. Rosie and I were given a bedroom to share.

The inhabitants of Hohwald gave us a great welcome on the evening of our arrival. Men, women and children in the national dress of Alsace danced and sang for us at the Auberge Eboué and we had plenty of *eau-de-vie* and sausages.

While the main hospital and the division rushed back to Alsace the remainder at Charentes was not idle. Colonel Mondain and Lieutenant Cappelle operated on the wounded brought in and supervised 180 beds. These were always full and stretchers sometimes had to be brought in as extra beds. There were many civilian casualties as well and several medical cases, some with diphtheria.

The German Admiral Kuetz, in command of the German lines, entered into negotiations with General de Larminat for medical aid and eventual evacuation of the civilian wounded. On 9 January a surgical team from Spears left the *Maison de Retraite* for the German lines. They were commanded by Colonel Mondain with Solly Albert, *sous officier* Cappelle and medical student Ceres, together with Sergeant Yantze, orderlies and Red Cross nurses, and as much medical equipment as could be packed into four hospital trucks. With Red Cross flags flying from each vehicle, they drove along a road mined on each side until they reached the first barricade. Here they were met by a German officer who escorted them through several more barricades until they reached the centre of Royan.

They set up a first-aid post and a clinic in the school, where the German authorities had assembled all the civilian casualties. Fifty were immediately sent to the hospital at Sainte and the lightly wounded treated on the spot and discharged to their homes. One baby was delivered.

In all, a total of 200 civilians were evacuated to Spears; the German wounded were looked after by their own doctors. The return of the unit to Sainte was made under the same conditions as their departure. They returned on 10 January, three hours before the truce ran out.

It was a curious experience for those taking part. They said the Germans behaved correctly and gave all the help they could. The German officer who assisted the team expressed surprise at the skill and quality of our medical officers, and was very impressed by the quality of the medical equipment, saying it was much superior to their own. The unit related many experiences and returned with a quantity of loot and presents – some legal, some not.

On 12 January they received orders to pack up and to join the main hospital as soon as possible. They arrived at Hohwald on 26 January and the hospital was together again.

The cold was intense throughout January and February, and we were very lucky to be billeted in the *Auberge Eboué*, which was always snug and well heated. With the help of our greatcoats and Canadian woollies we conserved the warmth we had built up inside the *auberge* for at least an hour when we were driving our cars.

By now our cars were very old indeed and, having been altered for the desert, had no interior heating. All of them had suffered from broken windows at one time or another and these had been replaced by ill-fitting plywood boards. There was no such thing as anti-freeze in those days and after each trip we had to drain the water from the pipes and radiators. Every time we set off we had to refill the radiators with hot water and quickly get the engines running before the water froze. The roads were deep in snow which meant fitting chains on the wheels before attempting the slightest incline. The chains had a very short life and were always breaking and as soon as we reached the top of a hill we had to get out and take them off again. It was a wearisome task, with wet and ice-cold fingers, making every journey twice as long as normal. A broken chain on one of the back wheels could cut straight through the rubber filling tube to the petrol tank and even hole the petrol tank itself. It was difficult to spot a broken chain before it had done the damage without continually getting out of the car to look.

We bartered bully beef and spam for bottles of kirsch and schnapps, which we kept hidden under our driving seats, and the *eau de vie* was a great help in keeping the cold at bay – no such thing as the breathalyser in those days!

When we had a few hours off duty we would ski on a slope opposite the main hospital. Someone managed to collect some skis and the beginners, including me, were initiated into the rudiments of skiing by Capitaine La Baume of the Foreign Legion who, before the war, had been an officer in the Chasseurs Alpins. He taught us to ski in the approved army fashion, standing erect as we whizzed down the slope. I was doing quite well until one day I hit a mole hill at speed and did half a dozen somersaults. I lost my confidence.

11 January – The hospital filled up with wounded and I was back nursing again. I was put in charge of 50 light cases housed on a floor at the top of the hotel which consisted of a series of small rooms with three or four beds in each room, except for one which was larger and had a balcony attached to it.

I had some very strange patients, including several goumiers from Morocco, civilian as well as military, with frost-bitten fingers and toes. There were also several women, including a Moroccan prostitute from the goum travelling brothel. She had third degree burns on her face, arms and legs, the result of lighting a fire with petrol that flashed back at her. I had to keep her alone with her door firmly locked after finding her terrified by three goumiers competing for her favours. She was a picturesque sight with her hennaed hair, bright green satin trousers and richly embroidered jacket.

In the larger room my patients consisted of a French ATS suffering the effects of a miscarriage and haemorrhage, and a very badly wounded mother with her small daughter who was unhurt. The most difficult patient of all was the Mother Superior of a nearby convent who had been caught in the crossfire of an attack. She was wounded in both legs and one arm. She complained bitterly at having to share a room with the other women, and was particularly unchristian to the small girl who was a good little thing and gave no trouble but, like all children, was inquisitive and at times noisy.

The nun did her utmost to persuade the Colonel to put her in a room of her own, but the only single room was occupied by the Moroccan woman who could not be moved. I told the Colonel that if the Mother Superior was the Virgin Mary herself I would still be unable to give her a room. He laughed and did not insist. I did compromise by putting screens round her bed and forbade the child to peep through them. We sent her back to the convent as soon as she was well enough to be moved.

Our division was holding a front of some 54 kilometres and this, in spite of the loss of a great many vehicles from tanks to trucks – many written off during the double journey through France – and more materiel they had been obliged to leave with the West Atlantic Division for their attack against the pocket at Royan.

The division was only able to send a few patrols over the Rhine and we were forced to abandon the villages of Gersthein, Oberheim and Hersherm, among others, owing to the pressure of enemy attacks and of the necessity to defend Strasbourg to the last. It was touch and go until help arrived.

As the bitter fighting for Strasbourg continued, Hohwald was flooded with the passage of civilian refugees who were fleeing from the city and the surrounding towns and villages. Little groups of people were heading for the centre of France, crossing the snow-covered countryside in the bitter cold. Many of them halted for a night's rest at Hohwald before continuing their trek, and we helped them when we could with food and shelter.

Plans were made for the evacuation of the hospital and its personnel if Strasbourg fell. I don't think we really believed it would and had very little time to listen to rumours or speculations. It never entered our heads that our division, which had triumphed so magnificently all the way up the desert and in Italy and France, could possibly be beaten.

Between 9 January and 6 March we admitted 1,880 patients – at least 20 a day and once as many as 84. At one time we had 400 patients with equipment and facilities for only 200 beds.

A large proportion of officers were among the wounded and 26 died in hospital and were buried in the divisional cemetery at Obernai. Their graves were dug by German prisoners, who had great difficulty in penetrating the frozen snow and ground.

Colmar was liberated on 2 February and the whole of Alsace was freed from the Germans six days later. Everywhere Alsatians, wearing national dress, celebrated.

The new German plastic mines, which were undetectable under several feet of snow and ice, caused considerable civilian and military casualties and once the fighting had ended we had a steady stream of officers and men requiring old wounds to be looked at and the odd bullet and shrapnel to be removed.

My cramped rooms at the top of the hotel were filled to capacity with 65 patients who, except for the women, were mostly light cases. By the end of January most of them had been evacuated, including all the women, and I handed over the remainder to the 'Marionettes', as the soldiers called French auxiliary nurses. They had been recruited by the Colonel when we were so busy and were the cause of a rift in the unit when Lady Spears arrived.

20 January – Set off en mission with Bazooka as companion to Aix-en-Provence and Alès to try and persuade two of the Colonel's doctor friends to join the hospital staff, which was still short of surgeons. This mission turned out to be the longest and most accident-involved trip of my war career.

21 January – I set off in the morning, having collected some new chains, and fitted them on 82 as the roads were very bad, covered with

frozen snow and with many deep drifts. I came across many accidents caused by skidding and passed several trucks stuck deep in drifts. One held me up for an hour as convoys bottle-necked in each direction. Immediately I had got past this hold-up a GM skidded into me and knocked me into a drift, but luckily I was able to get out of it with a little help.

All the signposts were down and a blizzard began, blocking out everything. I lost my way several times but eventually reached Bourbon les Bains after dark and made a bee-line for my friends, the mayor and his wife. As always, they generously let me have a hot bath, dinner and a warm bed. The next morning I made an early start after a huge breakfast of bacon and eggs and hot croissants.

22 January – I reached Dijon at 11am. There was even more snow on the road and I stopped at Chalon for a hot (but not very good) meal. I arrived at Lyons at 3pm – it looked very different from when we had arrived on the day of its liberation – snow everywhere, the building grey and sombre and the pedestrians equally so. I made my way to Claridges Hotel and the proprietor and his wife also gave me a very warm welcome. I took 82 to a garage to have her cut-out seen to as it was behaving badly. I was back at the hotel in time for a large tea, and an even larger dinner, topped up with wine, champagne and brandy – another example of the generosity of ordinary French people when they had so little for themselves.

23 January – On leaving the hotel the next morning I filled up with petrol at an army depot, by which time the cut-out had cut out again. I found an American ordnance depot who repaired it for me, but it failed again after only an hour and all I could do was to continue and pray that my battery would not become completely flat.

I reached Aix at 3.30pm and drove straight to the first doctor's house and delivered the Colonel's message. The doctor refused to join the hospital but said he had a colleague whom he thought might accept and he would contact him and let me know the answer the following morning if I would take responsibility, to which I agreed.

I tried, unsuccessfully, to get my car serviced and repaired. I spent the night at an RAF officers' hostel.

24 January – An RAF officer took me to an army garage where, once again, they put my battery on charge while they mended my cut-out. The doctor's friend – Dr Long – telephoned to say he would accept the Colonel's offer after all and as soon as 82 was ready I collected him. I then drove on to Alès for the second doctor, who kept me hanging about while he made up his mind whether or not to return with me. He finally made the decision not to as he said his wife was ill.

At least I had collected one doctor for the Colonel which I hoped had made my journey worthwhile.

I made my way back to Vals les Bains by nightfall, along a road badly snowed up. I had to use the chains several times and Dr Long and I spent the night in a comfortable *auberge*.

25 January – We set off for Le Chambon to see the Colonel's children and deliver presents from him. We drove along narrow mountainous roads, with snow becoming deeper and ever increasing snow drifts. We kept the chains on all the wheels but kept on getting stuck. Finally we came to a crossroads which was completely blocked and we had to retrace our steps to the main road to Le Chambon. This time I got through, reaching Le Chambon at tea time. I collected the children from their various schools and gave them their presents. I set off again for St Etienne where my passenger had friends who fed us and put us up for the night.

26 January – Reached Lyons at 9.30am and set off to the French *Sixième Bureau* to persuade them to give me the necessary papers to obtain a new set of tyres for Buzz. I collected the tyres from a French army garage and then went to an American depot where they fitted a new cut-out and petrol pump for me. We had an excellent lunch at a black market restaurant and I collected Marie le Mâitre, one of the French girls, who had joined us in Tunisia and who had been in hospital there.

We eventually left Lyons late in the afternoon but were held up for a long time not far from the centre by a tree which had fallen across the road. It had to be chopped up and dragged away before we could get through and we did not reach Dijon until well after dark. I had to drive the last forty miles without any lights. I had great difficulty finding rooms for the three of us so late at night. In the end Marie and I stayed in an American nurses' hostel and Dr Long stayed with some of his friends.

27 January – A very heavy fall of snow during the night made if difficult to reach the garage where I had left 82 for the night. I had to walk through snow up to my knees and got very wet. When I reached 82 it was even more difficult to dig a way out for her and then to collect Dr Long through more roads deep in snow.

The roads had been even more precarious but I managed to reach the small town of Langres without using my chains which, by this time, had become very thin. In the centre of Langres I got completely stuck as the inhabitants had shovelled the snow from the outside of their houses into the middle of the street. It took the combined efforts of two GMCs, one pulling and the other pushing, to get me out. The officer in charge of the trucks gave me a new set of chains and helped me to put them on. He told me that the road to Épinal was completely blocked by snow, but as it was the only road back I had no alternative but to take it.

As there were no inclines in the road I took off my chains as I didn't dare risk using them for long periods. I immediately skidded into a drift but managed, somehow, to get out again under my own steam. Then I skidded into a tree when trying to avoid a jeep which was skidding towards me. I had to be pulled out by another GMC.

Another six miles on and I was stuck again. Yet another GMC came to my rescue and towed me for ten miles along a terrible road rutted by the heavy trucks and tanks which made it impossible for a light staff car.

After the GMC had unhooked me I put the chains back on again. The road began to improve and eventually we reached Épinal. A one-way track had been dug through the snow, which was fine until we met another vehicle. When this happened it meant either backing to a passing place or digging a passage through, which was exhausting and time-consuming.

At Épinal I found that one of the chains had broken and cut through the rubber petrol filling tube. Fortunately I found a very helpful American garage whose sergeant not only promised to have it mended for me by the morning but found rooms for us all for the night. Marie and I had to share not only a bedroom but also a bed, so neither of us got much sleep.

28 January – The car was mended by 9am. Not only had the petrol pipe been cut in two but the petrol tank was full of a mixture of petrol, snow and water and had to be drained and cleaned.

The roads were snow-bound and our progress very slow; I had to make several detours before we reached St Martin at midday. I tried to go the shorter way to Hohwald along a hilly secondary road and got in a drift once again, which I was unable to get out of. This time I had to walk two miles down the road before I could get help. A divisional GMC came to my aid, but as it was pulling me out it pulled off the radiator tap and all the water ran out. I had to be towed to the Atelier Lourd for them to mend it. While it was being repaired the officers gave us a welcome hot meal.

We set off on the last lap of the journey as it was getting dark. We had only 30 kilometres to go but were held up several times by blockages and finally by a civilian car stuck in the middle of the road. As it proved to be immovable, I had no alternative but to retrace my steps and try another road. By this time it was completely dark and I still had no lights. Very fortunately we caught up with Germaine Sablon who guided me the last few miles with the lights of her car. I decanted my passengers and then had to dig a way through the snow into our garage before I could house 82. At last I tottered into the Auberge Eboué wondering whether I would ever feel warm again. After a welcome hot bath I snuggled down in bed.

Lady Spears and Dorea Stanhope had arrived at the hospital while I was away and La Générale was in high dudgeon over the increased size of the hospital – 400 beds instead of the agreed 200 – and the necessary influx of personnel, orderlies, doctors and female aides recruited to look after them. It was above all the female staff which infuriated her the most. Everywhere she went she came across strange women recruited by the Colonel. These women refused to take orders from Jean Barr, our very capable and popular Head Sister. The patients complained that the high standard of nursing they had come to expect from 'Spears' had fallen and the hospital was no longer the happy working unit it had always been.

Franka Cohen, the Theatre Sister, was particularly incensed by strange French women who appeared at intervals in her theatre, gave an anaesthetic or two for a strange new doctor, created minor chaos and then disappeared, leaving her to clear up the mess.

The sisters were all in a state of revolt and we, the drivers, backed them. Jean and her husband Pat gave in their notice. Jean said that she could not be responsible for the lives of the patients without the corresponding authority over the nursing staff. Kit and I also handed in our notice, in support of Jean, but Lady Spears refused to accept them.

There was also trouble over the name of the hospital, which hurt Lady Spears deeply. General de Gaulle, who had a personal hatred of General Spears after the troubles in Syria, where General Spears was the British representative had sent an order to the divisional HQ. The name 'Hadfield–Spears' was to be changed to HCM – Hôpital Chirurgical Militaire. Lady Spears rushed off to see General Garbay who, according to her, was all sympathy and ignorance. He sent her to see General Geurriac, Inspector of the French Army Service de Santé, who also expressed sympathy but denied all knowledge of the order. He gave Lady Spears permission to have a new stamp made with Ambulance Hadfield–Spears printed under the title HCM. Lady Spears returned triumphant and reported her success to the Colonel who exploded with rage and told her that both the Generals had lied to her. He showed her the order which stated plainly that – after visiting the Hospital – General de Lattre and Monsieur Diethelm (Minister for War for de Gaulle) had given instructions for the hospital to be renamed HCM and the name 'Spears' omitted! This order had been signed by Geurriac and carried his official stamp. However, Lady

Spears had won the day, and the new stamp was ordered and used until the end of the war.

During the following weeks the high feelings in the unit over the 'foreign invasion' ebbed and flowed. Jean and Pat left in the end and Lady Spears, with her usual tact and firmness, smoothed out the most serious wrinkles. The worst offenders were transferred and the remainder accepted with the increased size of the hospital. Although the hospital never quite regained its old familiar atmosphere it did retrieve its efficiency and continued as the competent machine it had always been.

Once Alsace had been liberated we went on several sightseeing tours. I fell in love with Strasbourg, the capital, bordered by the river Rhine. There was lots to see – the town was full of old black and white buildings, cobbled streets and a magnificent cathedral.

9 February – I did the post in Jean's jeep which someone had given to her, and she christened *Au Poil*, an appropriate name. I had a puncture outside HQ and no spare wheel so I stopped for lunch while it was mended. Rosie, Kit and I drove off in Buzz to spend the day with the Fusiliers Marins. After lunch in their mess we watched a review of René's squadron by their Colonel and then set off in two jeeps to inspect the front line. We climbed up into an observation post in a derelict house at Rhineau and peeped across the Rhine through broken windows. We failed to see any Germans moving around although we saw their dug-in tanks and field guns quite plainly.

10 February – Mrs Benson, who was head of the American relief fund, arrived to inspect the hospital. We hoped that she would allot to us sufficient funds to replace our worn-out trucks and equipment and perhaps even a staff car or two.

12 February – I was detailed to drive Mrs Benson to Paris and to take Jocelyn as well for her home leave. We set off after a night of torrential rain; there were floods everywhere and water rushing down the roads. 82 had lost her windscreen wipers which meant frequent stops to clear off the mud flung up by the heavy lorries. We reached Paris in good time, having stopped for a few minutes at Nancy and had lunch from our rations. We dropped Mrs Benson at the American Embassy and I went to SHAEF and the British Embassy to arrange our billets and a pass to England for Jocelyn. 82 had no lights and I was thankful to park her before I ran into something. I managed to get a double room at the Bedford Hotel for Jocelyn and myself.

13 February – I contacted Iris who was stuck in Paris, hoping to persuade the British workshops to mend 76 for her. They repaired the lights on 82 and gave me a new set of windscreen wipers.

14 February – I returned to Hohwald alone and had three punctures on the way, then a burst tyre which was caused by a broken wheel hub cutting through the tyre. I was able to scrounge a jeep wheel and tyre from a USA base camp. I fitted the hub screws but, as the wheel was smaller than 82's other wheels, it made the steering unsteady, but it got me back.

16 February – I drove Lady Spears to visit the concentration and extermination camp at Struthof. The camp was situated in the centre of pine-covered hills overlooking the plains of Alsace. 20,000 women and children had perished there. The Commandant of the camp lived in a small hotel belonging to Madame Eboué, who came with us. Her niece lived on a farm below the camp and supplied it with turnips and potatoes.

We were shown over the camp by a French officer who was in charge of several hundred German and Alsatian women. The former were accused of torture and sadism, the latter of collaboration with the Germans. We were shown the gas chamber where thousands of women and children had been suffocated. It had a tiled floor and walls, all in white, but no windows. It looked like a gigantic wash room, spotlessly clean. It was hard to imagine what had taken place there; only a short while before women and children had stood, stripped naked with their heads shorn. We were shown a whip with which one of the German commandants had whipped 400 women to death. Apparently he went mad in the end. This same commandant had planted a vegetable garden on the perimeter of the camp which he fertilised with bone meal from the incinerator, small white slivers which were still to be seen on the ground. We were shown parchment lamp shades which we were told were made out of human skin.

As we drove away down the winding road to have tea with Madame Eboué's niece we met a column of women returning from their walk. Their guards made them kneel down on the road with their heads bowed, which struck me as unnecessary but the hatred and brutality in some of their faces was frightening. We were amazed to see that several of the women were smartly dressed in beautiful fur coats, elegant shoes, silk stockings and stylish hats. They looked well nourished; many had sullen faces and glared at us with hate in their eyes.

Lady Spears asked Madame Eboué's niece if they had known what was happening in the camp. 'Oh yes!' she said. They had heard terrible screams day and night, and had seen many corpses when they delivered their vegetables. But, she asked, what could they do, as they were in fear of losing their own lives as well. In the end they just shut their ears to the screams and tried not to see the hands held out for food.

Lady Spears and I both found it difficult to swallow the tea we were offered and impossible to eat the cakes after the horror stories we had been told. I did not sleep for several nights afterwards.

20 February – The Foreign Legion, who had been very concerned about the troubles in the hospital and, above all, over the change of its name, arranged a dinner party in their mess in honour of Lady Spears. They wanted to impress upon her the strength of their solidarity and their appreciation for all she had done for the division with her Ambulance unit. Colonel de Lange was our host and the dinner ended with an enormous cake with 'Spears' written on it in icing. Emotional speeches and songs in French and English followed and, of course, the Legion's own song *Le Boudin* (Black Pudding).

28 February – René and the Fusiliers Marins invited Rosie and me, who were given a day off, to a magnificent banquet in the German Emperor's hunting lodge at Haut Königsburg, a fairy-tale castle perched on top of a mountain overlooking the Black Forest. The narrow road leading up to it wound its way round and round the mountain like a corkscrew. The castle, topped with towers and turrets, was filled with ancient armour and weapons and its walls hung with hunting trophies.

The festivities started early in the morning with a Catholic service taken by all the Padres of the division in the castle chapel, which until then had only had Protestant services held in it. This was followed by brass bands playing Alsatian songs, accompanied by girls in Alsatian national dress singing and dancing while we sipped white wine. After this everyone took part in 'La Chasse' in the surrounding woods. I don't think any game was shot but there was a lot of noise and shouting.

We returned to the château at lunch time and sat down to a banquet in the chevaliers' hall. The table was decorated with boars' heads, huge hams and giant dishes of various meats. While we ate a band played in the minstrels' gallery.

On our return to the hospital we found Iris had come back from Paris but without her car, 76. It had finally been declared unrepairable by the British workshop, who would not allow it out of their garage and lent her a truck to return to the hospital.

Orders arrived from HQ that the division was to be taken out of the line and sent to the South of France to mop up isolated pockets of

Germans firmly entrenched in pill-boxes strung along the Alpes Maritime between the frontier of France and Italy.

The division was very disappointed and bitter at not being allowed to cross the Rhine and continue the advance into Germany proper. Each regiment and unit in the division gave a party to celebrate the liberation of Alsace. We also gave a party and invited the senior officers of each unit. Charles Trenét and other French artistes came down from Paris to entertain the division, which was in great heart despite the disappointment at not reaching Germany.

16

THE LAST BATTLE

9 March 1945 – We left Hohwald at 6am and I drove Duprez to Roche, twelve miles from Besançon. I had to drive him round to find and allocate billets for everyone. Rosie and I were given a room with a single bed in it, which we had to share, in a cottage belonging to a kindly old peasant couple.

10 March – We travelled from Roche to Villebois. The snow had now disappeared and the temperature became noticeably warmer. The drivers were all lodged together in a small hotel with the promise of a day's rest, which our old cars needed, even if we did not. I had left 82 at the French Air Force Depot to be repaired.

12 March – The convoy left for Grenoble without Kit and me as 82 was not ready. We collected 82, ready washed and mended, and returned to Villebois where Schick had a splendid meal waiting for us – *hors d'oeuvre*, rabbit, omelette and strawberry tart followed by coffee. We left later and on reaching Grenoble found that everyone had been waiting for three hours for billets. We were finally allotted rooms in the Hotel Angleterre; it was very cold and the bed linen was dirty. It was not much warmer than at Hohwald but we did see primroses and violets along the roadside on our route. Denise, one of the French nurses, and Joan had been sent to the local hospital at Grenoble with measles. The Colonel had gone to Nice to make arrangements for the installation of the hospital. We ate a very bad supper at the *Poppette des Officiers* at Grenoble and Jocelyn and I went to the cinema to see a lamentable film called *Gunga Din*.

13 March – I went to a Ford garage to get a new spring for 82. I didn't have the time to get it fixed but at least I had succeeded in getting hold of a new one at long last. Rosie and I found a hairdresser and had our hair and faces cleaned. The Colonel returned and announced that he had found a good hotel in Nice where the hospital could be housed, so we prepared to leave the next day.

14 March – The main convoy left first thing in the morning. The staff cars, sisters and drivers remained in Grenoble for another day as the distance was only 300 kilometres, which we could do in a few hours. All our cars were serviced and ready so we were able to enjoy

ourselves. Kit and I drove up to a mountain peak to watch the sunset over the Alps.

15 March – We set off for Nice at 7am by the *Route Napoléon*. It was a lovely drive through the Alps, very hilly and twisty, bordered by pine trees covered with spiders' webs glistening in the early morning sunlight. The Colonel met us and sent us on to Cannes; we had to hang about for ages before we were installed in the Hôtel des Pins. The next day I took 82 to the Atelier Lourd to have her new spring fitted.

17 March – Left Cannes for Paris in Marguerite with Kit who was due for her fortnight's leave in England. My orders were to wait for Lady Spears, returning from London, and drive her back to the hospital.

Kit and I took it in turns to drive through the night. We reached Lyons at four in the morning and had some difficulty in finding petrol. Finally, we found an American depot which was open but unattended. We wandered round it shouting and sounding our horn and when we got no reply, we decided to help ourselves. We filled up Marguerite, and our petrol cans, and could not resist whipping a few brand new spanners and other tools which, we told each other, would come in useful for maintenance.

We reached Paris at midday and lunched at the British Officers' Club; I booked myself into the Bristol Hotel, the British Officers' transit camp. I helped Kit collect her papers and tickets for England and took her to the airport; then returned to the hotel and slept like a log until late the next morning. After lunch I went racing at Auteuil with an American officer friend of Major King and backed four winners out of five.

20 March – I met René's mother and took her to lunch at the *Club Interallie*, of which I was a member. It was a very smart club next to the British Embassy in the *Rue St Honoré* with a large garden and excellent food. Millet and Barbarot took me to visit the artist Ceci, who painted a portrait of Barbarot.

Cornelius, another Fusiliers Marins officer, took me to visit his father – another artist. There was great concern in his family as his brother had volunteered to fight with the Germans. Cornelius managed to get him sent to IndoChina later on.

Millet and Barbarot took me dancing at Ciro's Club and we had lunch with Cornelius and his family. They had a charming house and gardens.

I remained in Paris for thirteen days waiting for Lady Spears to return. Her arrival was postponed day by day. I didn't worry too much as I was having a happy time enjoying myself and meeting lots of friends from the Fusiliers Marins and Divisions. There was the dancing at Ciros and the Bal Tabarin, racing at Auteuil, and a Free French benevolent concert where Josephine Baker sang and de Gaulle was the guest of honour.

I did some work as well collecting new badges for the unit. I went to various HQs for the division and to Versailles to the British workshops, removing every possible spare part from Iris's condemned 76 which might be of use for our other cars. I also managed to persuade the officer in charge to give us three new Hillman staff cars as replacements for our old crocks and finally collected a large number of goods for the foyer Germaine Sablon ran for our wounded patients.

29 March – I collected Lady Spears, at last, at the Gare du Nord and took her to the Vendôme hotel, at the corner of the Place Vendôme. The next day I drove her all round Paris and invited her to lunch at the *Club Interallie*.

I dropped her off at her hotel and loaded up Marguerite with all the clobber I had collected to be ready for an early start. The next morning I picked up Lady Spears and we set off with her for Cannes. We stopped on the way at a small village near Avalon for her to visit a cemetery where the grandmother and other relations of General Spears had been buried. We lunched at Avalon and spent the night at the Hotel Claridge at Lyons. We were given my usual welcome and invited to dine with the proprietor and his wife.

During the journey Marguerite's steering became more and more eccentric. She would dive into the centre of the road without any warning, several times when I was passing another vehicle. Lady Spears, sitting in the back reading one of her detective novels as usual, noticed nothing, but I began to wonder whether we would reach Cannes without an accident or breakdown.

1 April – Reached Orange for lunch and from there took the Corniche road from Fréjus to Cannes. The hospital was still at the Hôtel des Pins but due to move to Beaulieu at midday the following day. The hospital was to be installed in the enormous Bristol Hotel, situated on the top of a hill overlooking the small town with splendid views over the houses and sea.

The hospital at Beaulieu was all on the ground floor. The large reception rooms made excellent wards and the sitting rooms and card rooms became operating theatres, X-ray, reception, *etc*. The staff were housed on the three upper floors, the women on the third.

We had the impression that we were experiencing the luxury of the very rich. Each of us had an enormous bedroom, and the luckier ones a suite. Each bedroom had its own bathroom, tiled from floor to ceiling in spotless white with a huge glistening bath tub with shining taps and a shower. Alas, no hot water, and often no water at all. Broken panes of glass let in the rain and the damp sea breezes – and the mistral, when it blew. Torn brocaded curtains flapped round the windows in the breezes. Plaster had fallen from the ceilings and the walls were cracked and peeling. Even so, we appreciated the space and grandeur and enjoyed imagining what sort of clientèle the hotel had welcomed in pre-war days. The warmth and beauty of the Côte d'Azur with all the mimosa and scented flowering shrubs was a welcome change from the ice and snow of Alsace.

Some of the units, and in particular the officers of the division, had succeeded in requisitioning empty villas on the Corniche and lived in great style with their private swimming pools and comfortable furniture – often with servants, under contract to their absent employers, to look after them.

3 April – I took Marguerite to a garage to find out why her steering was erratic. They found that the front axle was broken and the right-hand king pin, holding the track-rod, was completely worn through and hanging on by a thread. If it had broken off we might have had a serious accident.

4 April – Lady Spears took Jocelyn, Kelsey and I to a luncheon party at the Carlton Hotel in Cannes given by a princess she had known before the war. The other guests were all rich and rare cosmopolitans and – it appeared from their conversation – very remote from the reality of the war. We were shocked as they gave us the impression of not caring who won the war as long as they were able to continue their lives of pleasure and gaming.

Later, when the hospital was full of wounded, no one from outside came to visit the patients or showed the slightest interest in their well-being. This so enraged Germaine Sablon that she wrote a scathing letter to the local newspaper and they printed it on the front page. The response was immediate. Chauffeur-driven limousines rolled up with comforts and occasionally visits in person by rich dowagers.

One night I went to the casino at Monte Carlo with Germaine; it was run by her brother Jean, the singer. Rosie and René joined us; we had to wear civilian clothes as no one was allowed in wearing uniform. We wandered round the tables at the casino; I was fascinated by the faces of the many old crones playing roulette with their claw-like hands flashing over the table to collect the chips when they won. We were told that many of them had lived in Monte Carlo for most of their adult lives and they only came to life when the casino opened its doors. They arrived there every night and remained until the casino closed, compulsive gamblers with no other interest in life.

7 April – The division was in position to attack the Germans in the Alpes Maritime. The hospital sent off two forward units, one to Lantosque at the foot of l'Authion, which consisted of 60 beds and stretchers cramped into a tiny caverne which had been used before the war by the Chasseurs Alpins. The second unit was sent to St Etienne des Tinée, further north, and was installed in a small bistro with room for 30 beds and stretchers.

9 April – Lady Spears asked me if I would go up to the forward post at St Etienne and help with the nursing. I left the following morning in Buzz, having collected some PX rations from the Americans on the way. A lonely, twisty, beautiful road between the mountains and overlooked by the Germans in their pill-boxes, who amused themselves by taking pot shots at our vehicles, led to St Etienne.

On my arrival I found the last three patients had been evacuated that morning. There was nothing for me to do so I went to the nearby village and bought myself a fishing rod and tried, unsuccessfully, to catch a trout in the fast-running stream alongside the road. Lady Spears and Rosie turned up at the post for tea and I missed them.

It was very cold at St Etienne and it felt all the more so after the warmth of Beaulieu. There was no heating in the auberge and no fires and it was difficult to sleep at night under insufficient blankets. Luckily the sun shone strongly during the day and thawed us out.

We received only four patients and I began to get fed up with nothing to do. There were twelve of us to look after the four lightly wounded men. We spent our time fishing, unsuccessfully, or sitting out in the sun in front of the auberge playing cards or reading.

11 April – Still tired of nothing to do. Yantze and I went fishing with an old fisherman who caught dozens of trout; We only caught one each. The next day there was still no work so I drove to Aurès, about seven kilometres away, to look at the Olympic ski run. It was a pretty drive twisting through the Alps.

13 April – At tea time Jocelyn arrived to replace me, with a message from Lady Spears saying she wanted me to return immediately as they were desperately busy. Welcome news – I threw my things into Buzz and set off without a backward glance and, by 8pm, I was working in reception. The hospital was overflowing with wounded and in this, the last campaign of the division, we admitted 2,899 patients. Eleven died in hospital and many more in battle.

Many people thought this campaign was unnecessary, arguing that the Germans in their pill-boxes, sited in such a way that they were practically impregnable, except by frontal attack which ensured heavy casualties, would have surrendered anyway when the cease-fire was declared.

Others claimed that the Massif Central had, above all, a strategic value as it guarded Nice and the Côte d'Azure on the one side and on the other the Col de Tendre, Turin and Piedmont in Italy. De Gaulle argued that if France was to obtain the ratification of the Italian frontier, she had to occupy all the French-speaking villages with her troops. This, at least, was the reason given to the division for one of the costliest battles in killed and wounded it had endured during all its campaigns.

These deaths were the saddest of the war. So many of the casualties were men who had surmounted all sorts of hazards to join the Free French and were the survivors of such a small band of original volunteers, badly needed to help rebuild France at the end of the war. They had fought all the way up the desert, in Italy and France and now, at the very end of the war, had lost their lives.

Most of the terrain fought over was in the Massif Central de Mercantour where the élite German 34th Division was firmly entrenched in the snow-covered mountain tops. Each stronghold was surrounded by every type of mine, including a new Italian personnel mine which was encased in wood and impossible to detect by mine detectors. These mines caused terrible wounds to body and limbs and permanently blinded many of our soldiers.

The division was aided not only by the French Maquis, who had fled to the mountains to escape being enlisted into the German army, but also by various brigades of Italian patriots, mainly the Guistizia, the Libetta and the Garibaldi. The first two wore bright green scarves and the last dark green jackets, and had been equipped by the SOE.

The territory was some of the most difficult the division had encountered. To allow the light tanks and guns to reach a firing position snow had to be bulldozed from the narrow tracks, which then had to be widened and cleared of mines and were always under attack from the German positions above.

The descent of the wounded was extremely arduous and distressing, often by mule and, in some cases, taking three days to reach our forward units. Many died from exposure and lack of medical aid on the way down, particularly the abdominal and amputation cases.

23 April – There were two almighty explosions in the small harbour of Beaulieu at 2am. The hotel shook and all the remaining glass in the windows blew in. In the morning we learnt that a German torpedo boat with a crew of four had entered the harbour. They had mistaken it for Villefrance, where several warships were at anchor, and fired their torpedoes. One of the Germans had been killed, one escaped and two others were taken prisoner and brought to the hospital. Each man was

encased in a black rubber suit, complete with flippers on their feet and diving masks on their heads. We were intrigued, as we had never seen anything like this before.

25 April – I was back driving again and drove Lady Spears for a trip to Monte Carlo and to Eze-sur-Mer, where her sister owned a house. Eze was a small village perched on the top of a rocky hill, with an uninterrupted view over the Mediterranean and cobbled streets, too narrow for cars or carts. It was very old and *classée* – which meant no old houses could be pulled down or new ones built. Some of the houses were built into the rocks. The house belonging to Lady Spears' sister, who was married to a Hungarian musician, was on two sides of the street with a bridge connecting the two parts on the first floor. They both escaped to the USA when the Germans overran France. We found it unharmed due to the devotion of the caretaker and his wife, who told us proudly that they had hidden all the silver and valuables and the wine from the Germans. Lady Spears decided to give a party in her sister's house at the weekend, which we all enjoyed.

The South of France was very short of food and communication with the rest of France almost non-existent. Few, if any, of the telephones were working. The railway had either been blown up by the Resistance or bombed by the RAF. The rolling stock had gone the same way or had been requisitioned by the Germans. The civilian population had virtually no petrol or lorries and there was great difficulty in transporting any food. On the roads one met the strangest vehicles which were running on gas made from vines or manure or wood. These curious machines had enormous balloons on their roofs, or stoves built on their rears.

Apart from fruit, vegetables and fish, very little else was produced in the South – no meat or dairy products. There was the odd raid into Italy and elsewhere; one night two cows appeared mysteriously in the garden of our hotel and for a week we all had fresh meat.

I had a small windfall at this time. A group of British officers, who had been seconded to the Italian patriots, were recalled to their units and gave me their surplus British rations. The trucks arrived with over five tons of bully beef, dried milk, cheese, jam, tea, coffee, sugar and soap. Rosie and I had a lucrative time swopping tins of bully beef and spam for silk underclothes in Monte Carlo until we flooded the market.

Bob Bentley, whom we had met at Zuara, near Tripoli, had been parachuted into Italy by the SOE to contact and help the Italian Resistance; he turned up one day and made me a present of several thousand lira which he no longer needed.

My problem then was how to spend it, as Italy was out of bounds to all troops. The frontier was heavily guarded by American Military

Police and I tried several times, without success. Kit had a bright idea of writing out an *ordre de mission* for ourselves. We managed to get hold of some lettered hospital paper and signed it Alison Smith (Colonel) – a name Kit thought up on the spur on the moment. We 'borrowed' the hospital seal, stamped it over the signature, and tried the frontier again.

This time, to our delight and surprise, we sailed through all the barriers without any trouble at all. We drove along a really frightening coastal road dug out of the cliffs, with crumbling sides falling sheer to the rocks and sea below. It was just wide enough for a car. Along one stretch of road the side had fallen away and there did not appear to be enough room for even Buzz to get by. Kit got out and directed me, inch by inch, until we were over it. We then passed through fields and fields of roses and carnations all in bloom which we stopped to pick and we bought silk garlands, Parma ham and butter with my lira.

1 May – With our *ordre de mission* still intact Kit and I set off for a second visit to Italy, this time to Imperia where Bob Bentley invited us to watch the victory parades of the patriots celebrating the liberation of Italy. We sat on a balcony overlooking the main square among the Imperia notables who were taking the salute. When it ended, Bob took us for a tour of Imperia which ended in a visit to the house of the famous clown, Grock. Grock had ordered his house to be unlike any other house in the world. It was decorated inside and outside with monstrous masks of himself. He was an ardent admirer of Hitler and the Nazis, so Kit and I had no qualms about taking a souvenir each. Kit chose a delightful metal model of a sleeping fox which was inscribed underneath as being a present to Grock from Goering in memory of a visit to Germany by the clown. I collected two small silvered elephants. The US army crossed the Brenner pass into Italy.

8 May – Mr Churchill announced peace in Europe. We heard his broadcast over the wireless at 3pm and all went into Nice. The division had a small parade, followed by a battery of gunfire. All night people danced in the streets.

There was a feeling of anti-climax in the division and among ourselves and our friends. We had lived from day to day with death just around the corner for so long; no one planned ahead as there did not seem to be any point. Now we were all to be plunged into civilian life, willy-nilly, earning a living, competing for jobs, and few of us enjoyed the prospect. After five years of war it would be a difficult change-over.

The last battle of the division had cost 273 dead and 744 grands mutilés de guerre – a very high price to pay for the honour of France. The last soldier to die of wounds in our hospital was Quartermaster

Combaz, who had lost both his legs when a mine exploded on 4 May; he died a week later.

Until all our patients had been evacuated we had a succession of distinguished visitors: General Doyen, commander of the Alp Army; General Garbay who inspected the personnel of the hospital and gave out a few medals; the Princess de Bearharnais, and many others.

Lady Diana Cooper, who was a friend of Lady Spears, and whose husband was the British Ambassador in Paris, arrived with her son, a boy of about twelve years old, to visit the Hospital. She was presented with a bouquet of flowers by the Colonel. When she arrived at the ward on which I was working she kept leaving the flowers on various patients' beds; each time they were rescued and given back to her. I was at the end of the ward near the exit renewing the dressings on a very young French boy who had lost both his legs. These dressings could not be done quickly, and however careful you were you could not avoid causing pain. The boy was desperate that Lady Diana should not see his stumps and kept telling me to hurry up. I told him not to worry, and if I had not finished I would cover him up with the sheet when she arrived. When Lady Diana arrived she asked me what the boy's wounds were. I told her, she smiled at him and said something encouraging and left her bouquet on his bed. This time it was not noticed, or perhaps her escorts were tired of rescuing it. The boy was so delighted; he said to me: 'There, you see the British ambassadress is a kind lady and was sorry for me so she left me her flowers'. I found a jar to put them in and arranged them on his bedside table. I didn't have the heart to tell him what I thought of Lady Diana.

After Germaine's letter to the local papers the indifferent local population woke up to the losses suffered by Frenchmen for Frenchmen. Some offered themselves as blood donors, while others organised parties of singers and entertainers to amuse the wounded. Many sent in gifts of flowers, fruit and food.

We should have been more grateful than we were, accepting rather than refusing the many invitations we, the English personnel, received to wine and dine with well-wishers. We probably would have done so if the casualties had not been so heavy but, after watching the ambulances unloading gravely-injured soldiers day after day, many of them our friends from the desert days, some already dead on their stretchers, others dying before they reached the operating tables, others maimed for life, we preferred to spend the last days of the war with our comrades in the division whom we knew so well and who shared our thoughts and unhappiness.

On my day off, La Lande and La Baume called in to see one of their wounded and I showed them the ward. Later I drove René to Grasse in Buzz where we saw the fields of lavender and other scented flowers. We visited a scent factory and smelt all the different aromas which were blended together to produce the expensive perfumes. We lunched there and then drove to Cannes through the mountains.

Major King turned up again, ostensibly to see if the cars had arrived okay. Lady Spears gave a party for him at Eze. He was very heavy and serious and seemed to have taken a liking to me, which was ridiculous. He was twice my age and had a perfectly good wife and daughter at home in England; moreover, he bored me to distraction. But May insisted that I be nice to him as it was because of him we had the new cars.

10 May – Rosie and I were given the weekend off. We had an invitation from Madame Fournier who owned Pourquerolle, an island off the coast of the Mediterranean, to join her there. We picked her up at Brignolles and went to Hyères where we met up with Millet and Barbarot, whom she had also invited. We crossed over to the island in an American MTB. We stayed as the guests of Madame Fournier in a small hotel on the shore of the island and swam, sunbathed and went for walks. We ate delicious fish dishes – langouste, crab, scampi, *etc*. The island was tiny with a few fishermen's cottages along the shore; very sparsely vegetated, a few pine trees and aromatic shrubs. It had a pill-box and a lighthouse, sandy beaches, a few sea birds but little else. We left on Monday morning and were back at Beaulieu at midday.

17 May – I drove René into Italy in Buzz with my *ordre de mission* to buy more supplies with my lira. A very pretty Italian girl came up and asked if I was English. I said I was; she said: 'I'm so glad. We Italians like the British but dislike the French intensely.' René's reply was unrepeatable.

During these last few days at Beaulieu, when there was very little driving or nursing, Rosie and I made friends with a French pilot who flew Piper Cubs – spotter planes – for the artillery. He offered to teach us both how to fly them. We had several lessons and were getting on really well when Lady Spears heard about it and forbade us to have any more lessons. This was odd as she was very seldom interfered with our private lives and went on the principle that 'it didn't matter what we did as long as we didn't frighten the horses'.

Rosie and I made last-minute dashes to Monte Carlo to collect the expensive underwear we had ordered; we paid for it out of the army rations I had been given.

1 June – The last hospital party – a *Bal Costumé* – was given by the Colonel and organised by Duprez. The fancy dress clothes and a band were hired from Monte Carlo. I was one of the last to collect a costume and all I could find was an Indian sari. Most of Beaulieu

gate-crashed the party and there was such a crowd of unknown people that I left at midnight.

The following day one of the trucks caught fire inside and the Colonel, extremely proud of himself, went round telling everyone that he had put it out by himself by peeing on it.

The Colonel had persuaded Lady Spears to offer the hospital to General de Gaulle for service in the Far East, where the war continued. We could provide a 100-bedded hospital on wheels by selecting the best of the material. There was no lack of volunteers to accompany it.

We left Beaulieu on 5 June with the rest of the division – 750 vehicles in all. I led our convoy, driving Lady Spears in a splendid Buick which someone had found hidden in a garage in Nice and presented to us.

The first night in convoy we halted near Aix, and the following morning I left the convoy with Lady Spears to visit Avignon and the Pope's palace. We caught up again near Lyons where we stopped for the night.

7 June – I drove Lady Spears, with Edith, to Paris. On the way, when we were doing 80 mph, the Buick had a burst front tyre. It felt as if the whole transmission had disintegrated and I had the greatest difficulty in holding the car on the road. We missed, only by inches, a white horse pulling a cart. Fortunately, the road had a slight incline which eventually slowed us up. I had turned off the ignition but did not dare to touch the brakes as we skidded from one side of the road to the other. There was an awful smell of burning rubber and the car crawled to a halt a few feet from a ditch.

My arms were aching from the effort of holding the car on the road and I was trembling all over. Lady Spears was quite unconcerned and merely said: 'This is how people get killed'. I stammered: 'Yes, you have just lost one of your seven lives.' When I examined the tyre, which was in shreds, I noticed that both wheels were out of alignment and the other front tyre was completely worn down to the canvas. With the help of the Colonel's wheel jack, as well as my own, we managed to change the back wheels to the front and, with the good spare wheel and succeeded in reaching Paris without further mishap. I took the precaution of driving much slower and inspected the tyres every 50 kilometres.

We spent the night at the Hotel Vendôme and next morning I drove Lady Spears to various bureaux and then left her at the British Embassy while I went to the British workshops at Versailles to wangle a set of new tyres, and to see if they could align the wheels for me. They put the Buick up on a ramp and we could see quite plainly that the whole of the chassis was cracked and irreparable. They very kindly lent me a staff car until one of our own arrived.

10 June – I drove Lady Spears to Trilport, a small village near Meaux. The hospital was opened for the last time. The barracks, containing 100 beds, was supplemented by one tent to ensure that the division was looked after until it was disbanded.

Cecil King took Lady Spears and me to lunch at the Meurice Hotel, after which I took her to Trilport where I remained. Iris, Kit and Rosie were already installed there; we were all lodged in an empty villa which was isolated from other buildings and the hospital. Rosie and I had dinner with René, Barbarot and a Colonel friend of theirs at an auberge belonging to one of René's petty officers. We were given an excellent meal which included an enormous omelette followed by strawberries and cream and I ate brie for the first time in my life. Another evening René arrived with a whole brie the size of a cartwheel for Rosie and me and then proceeded to eat nearly all of it himself.

Between the 12 and 23 June, we admitted 130 medical cases and 17 surgical, mostly motor accidents. Happily there were no deaths.

During the last days of May we learnt that fighting had broken out between the French Garrisons in Syria and the Syrians. The British troops, under General Paget, had to be called in to end it. General de Gaulle blamed General Spears and accused him of employing secret agents who had engineered the outbreak. The accusations and denials continued to the end of their lives.

The victory parade in Paris had been arranged by General de Gaulle for 18 June. This was to commemorate his famous appeal from London to France in 1940 which ended with the words: '*La France a perdu une bataille mais pas la guerre!*'

Because of the bad feeling between General Spears and General de Gaulle, Lady Spears went to see the British Ambassador to ask his advice on whether or not we should take part in the parade. Duff Cooper was quite adamant that we were all to take part and that we were to fly the Union Jack as well as the Tricolour. General Garbay and the division were also insistent that we should be part of the parade.

Meanwhile, at the hospital, we knew nothing of Lady Spears' hesitation and were working flat out for the great day. The FAU had to find six trucks out of their old crocks which would not let them down by collapsing half way down the Champs Elysées, and we had to choose four cars to carry us and the sisters through the parade as well. We repainted them all with the hospital flag picked out in bright colours. The design incorporated both flags and had been approved by de Gaulle when the hospital was formed. We cleaned and polished the cars until they shone. Our uniforms were cleaned and pressed and Sam Browne belts and buttons polished. We had never looked so smart. At the last minute we painted the car tyres white. We were given two small pennants to be flown from the staff cars, the French flag in the place on honour on the right hand side; the British flag on the left. Our place in the parade was assigned to us and we had one practice with the staff cars on a disused aerodrome – driving four abreast at 10mph.

18 June – We got up at 4am and left in convoy an hour later. As every driver wanted to drive in the parade I volunteered to go as a passenger with Lady Spears and Irving, with Kit driving us in the smart Graham–Page. Half way to Paris the Graham Page stalled. We were being towed to try and start her again when black smoke began to pour out of her undercarriage where a small fire had started. We managed to put it out before any serious damage was done. With the help, once again, of the Atelier Lourd we found the trouble and it was quickly repaired.

We all reached the Avenue de Grande Armée by 8am and found our place in the parade. A two-hour wait gave us time to buy croissants and a cup of coffee from a bistro. We used the lavatory in the bistro – a very primitive affair considering that it was in the middle of Paris – just a privy behind a broken door in a small courtyard.

It was midday before we finally moved off under a cloudless blue sky. The great avenues were crowded with spectators who were kept in line by police and soldiers while aircraft zoomed overhead in strict formation.

The Colonel led our group in a jeep with Nocetto, our Sergeant Major, beside him carrying high the banner given to us by the division, beautifully embroidered in white satin. The four staff cars followed the Colonel, flanked on each side by a jeep; then the six trucks driven by the FAU carrying our NCOs and orderlies. Our orders were to divide when we reached the Place de la Concorde where General Koenig would be standing – three vehicles to the right and three to the right – overlooked by de Gaulle who would take the salute with the Sultan of Morocco by his side.

We felt very proud and honoured to be taking part in this procession of the Free French Army in the capital of France. We thought we looked quite smart. The drivers were in their best khaki uniforms and the sisters in their pretty grey and blue outfits and our splendid new flag and pennants were fluttering in the breeze.

The speed of the parade was most erratic. One moment we were racing down the Champs Elysées at 25mph and the next moment we had to slow down to 5mph which made it extremely difficult for the drivers to keep in line. When we reached the Place de la Concorde we heard the familiar cries of '*Voilà Spears*' and '*Vive Spears*' which brought tears to our eyes. We divided at Koenig's feet and, once out of the parade, made a bee-line to the French Officers' Club to have something to eat and to celebrate the miracle that not one of our vehicles had broken down in the parade.

While we were eating our lunch an unknown French officer, lunching at another table, very aggressively asked me what right I had to wear the Commando flash on my shoulder. I became extremely embarrassed and stammered that Colonel Bouvet had presented it to me and told me that I was to wear it when we landed in the South of France on D-Day minus two. He had given one to all seven of us and told us that we were officially in the Commandos. The officer looked surprised and said that I must be very proud to wear it. At this Lady Spears, who had been listening to the conversation, looked very annoyed and said: 'Not at all, the Commandos were very proud of her and her small unit' – whereupon the officer apologised profusely. We all had a good laugh after his departure.

20 June – At the hospital celebrations party, which Lady Spears missed for some reason, the Colonel announced a bombshell, dropped upon us by de Gaulle. The Ambulance was to be disbanded in 48 hours, the French personnel returned to various units and all the English to be repatriated immediately. The problem was that dozens of our grands blessés, who were now in the Val de Grace, the military hospital in Paris, had been brought to the parade by Koenig and seated in the grandstand around and behind de Gaulle and all the important personages taking part, so that they could watch their comrades in arms parading.

Quite naturally, seeing us – *their* hospital – approaching in a rather unsteady line, they gave us the encouragement they always did by shouting: '*Vive l'Ambulance Spears*' the only name we were known by in the division, in spite of de Gaulle trying to change it.

The hospital had nothing whatever to do with General Spears apart from the name. He had never visited the hospital or taken any interest in it. This was completely misunderstood by de Gaulle, who exploded into wrath and demanded of Koenig '*Qu'est que c'est ça? Le nom Spears en Paris et le drapeau anglais.*' Koenig attempted to explain but de Gaulle refused to listen and sent off the order the following day which came through to us from the French Army HQ.

The Colonel was so distressed that he told no one of the orders for 24 hours, refusing out of delicacy to tell Lady Spears. While she was away in Paris he made the hospital celebrations an excuse to get us all together and tell us exactly what had happened and why. He risked his career by telling all the regiments of the division as well and each of them reacted in its own way.

Barbarot, Tripier, René, and others from the Fusiliers Marins, marched into de Gaulle's office and flung their medals down on his desk. All the Fusiliers Marins gave a party for Lady Spears and for us at the French Officers' Club in Paris. The Foreign Legion gave a dinner party for us in their mess and all the officers of the division came to the hospital to bid us farewell and, most touching of all, the Foreign Legion sent their famous band to play the Legion songs to us the morning we left the hospital.

We learnt from the British Embassy that de Gaulle went even further with his rage, refusing to allow certain officers – René, Barbarot, La Lande and St Hilier – to receive the MCs and DSOs they had been awarded, which should have been presented to them by Duff Cooper at a special ceremony following the parade.

A petty story, and a sad one for all concerned, touching diplomatic levels and reaching the press with letters flying backwards and forwards between de Gaulle, Lady Spears and others, of course, it was impossible to disband in 48 hours for many reasons, the main one being that we had 100 patients in the wards.

Lady Spears and most of the English personnel left on 23 June. Kelsey volunteered to remain with the French nurses to supervise the orderly evacuation of the patients and Jocelyn stayed on as Lady Spears's representative to hand over officially all the medical equipment to the Colonel to be used as he thought best.

So we never went to the Far East as Lady Spears had intended. Who knows what might have happened had we done so? One thing is certain; it would only have deferred the day when we became civilians again and faced the most difficult task so far – settling back to a 'normal' life.

The wounded German prisoners of war we treated in our hospital during the desert war – whatever their rank – were treated exactly the same as our own wounded. They behaved very correctly and never complained – unlike the Italians who always made such a fuss that one never knew how badly or lightly they were wounded.

The German army under Rommel also behaved impeccably; they treated their PoWs correctly, and Rommel even informed our army of the names and ranks of all captured British soldiers.

The Italians behaved despicably in many ways. In the desert, they scattered booby traps disguised as thermos flasks and fountain pens, so we were warned never to pick up anything lying around. The Italians also left booby traps around their dead; this was when Italian PoWs were made to bury their own dead. I was told also – but was never able to confirm – that the Italians sometimes tied up dogs near their dead which, when released, set off a mine which killed both the dog and its rescuer.

Many of the British PoWs captured in the desert were sent to Italian PoW camps in Italy where they were very badly treated. Before Italy capitulated, one of the camps was mistakenly bombed by the RAF and set on fire; not only did the Italian guards refuse to help rescue the prisoners trapped inside, but they refused to give the uninjured prisoners any means of rescuing them.

When we were in Tunisia we were given some Italian PoWs to help with the hospital work, but they were absolutely useless and we sent them all back.

It was not until we reached France and learnt of the concentration and extermination camps, and met the survivors of torture, and saw with our own eyes the horrors committed by the Gestapo and SS that I began to hate the Germans.

We had five staff cars for which we, the drivers, were entirely responsible. There were four Fords (54, 60, 76 and 82) and a Chevrolet (96). They were also painted with the Croix de Lorraine and the Hadfield–Spears badge. We had our own cars to look after and drive, though we drove any of the others as necessary. Kit's car was 96, mine was 82, Jocelyn's 54, Iris's 76 and Rosie's 60. The windows – including the windscreen – were painted over in khaki with only a slit to see through. This was to prevent the reflection of the sun giving our position away to enemy aircraft. When the desert war was over we were able to remove the paint from the windscreens and windows, though most of the glass had disappeared from the windows and had been replaced by wood. All the cars were fitted with desert tyres which, as far as I can remember, they kept until the end of the war. These were twice the size of ordinary tyres and helped in the sand but taking them off and replacing them on the hubs was hard work to say the least; we had to balance the wheel on an oil drum and lever the tyre off with special tools. The most difficult part was to get the inner tube in without pinching it as the tyre was inflated.

Each car was fitted with a water condenser attached to the radiator, essential in the desert heat. This did help, but still did not prevent the radiator from boiling over when we had to drive slowly as in convoy.

In the desert, we carried sand track on the roofs and in France snow chains. We carried petrol cans in the boot, as well as spare water, half shafts – which the Fords were famous for breaking – spare petrol pumps and carburettors, spare wheels, spare tyre and tube, tools and tow rope. Each car had a wooden roof rack which was always piled high whenever we moved house. For some reason Kit had fitted lorry springs to Marguerite, which meant she needed bags of sand in the boot to keep her on the road when driven over pot holes and bumps.

The cars had all done a high mileage by the time I joined the unit. Their windscreen wipers had long disappeared and their indicators and horns had become very unreliable as had their handbrakes. By the end of the war each car had covered over 200,000 miles and the only original bits of them left were the chassis.

We spent a lot of time in the desert scouting for wrecked staff cars to pick clean, taking everything we could find. Our Fords, which were never intended to have their nuts and bolts unscrewed (all American parts are expendable) – could only boast their chassis as original. We never had both hand and foot brakes in working order and we always left our cars in gear when parked, just in case.

We all had some pretty lucky escapes. Brakes failed, steering wheels came away in our hands, tyres blew, track-rods broke. Miraculously no one was killed or even seriously injured during the whole of the war. Rosie had a lucky escape when one of her friends gave her a landmine as a souvenir. She put it in the boot of her car and forgot all about it. A few days later she drove Lady Spears from the desert to Beyrouth, and then took the car to a civilian garage to be serviced. When she went to collect it the following morning she was amazed to see the entire garage staff waiting for her in the street in a great state of excitement. The manager told her that she had a live mine in her car. Rosie did not believe him but as they would not let her take the car she had to get help from the army – who found that the mine was live and took it away and exploded it. The fact that Rosie had driven

Lady Spears, happily sitting in the back reading her detective novels, some 1,000 miles over bad roads and potholes with a landmine in the back was a sobering thought for all of us.

My old car, 82, was the only one to survive the war in one piece, although with few of her original parts except the chassis. She ended her life in IndoChina with our old friends the Thirteenth Demi-Brigade of the Foreign Legion on a mine which killed Colonel de Savigné, one of the Free French volunteers and one of the bravest officers in the division. René identified the wreckage many years later – I think on the road to Dalat.